WAITING FOR THE HEALER

Eamonn Sweeney

WAITING FOR THE HEALER

PICADOR

First published 1997 by Picador

an imprint of Macmillan Publishers Ltd
25 Eccleston Place, London SW1W 9NF
and Basingstoke

Associated companies throughout the world

ISBN 0 330 35029 3

A CIP catalogue record for this book is available from
the British Library

Typeset by CentraCet, Cambridge
Printed by Mackays of Chatham PLC, Chatham, Kent

To my mother

Acknowledgements

Thanks to my agent Pat Kavanagh and publisher Peter Straus for their faith and especially to my editor Rachel Heath for her work on the book. Thanks to my family for their support and to my friends Siobhan Cronin and Ronnie Bellew for their help.

Contents

One

God Needs Bouncers

I did everything for the best. Everyone does everything for the best. You do it and you think the best way is how it's going to turn out. That's how you mean it to turn out. But it just turns out like it wants to. That's how it is.

Maybe it was my fault. I could have just let things go and not cared about them. But what I wanted to do was the best thing. The right thing. And look what happens.

Can you put a start to anything? Maybe where it started was nine o'clock in the jacks of a pub in the Square Mile. Another London Tuesday.

Where the fuck are you, lad? And why? Armitage Shanks, according to the sign in front of me. Vitreous china. Great stuff. Never been to Asia before.

A lot of spit in the bowl. A few

lumps floating in it. No big deal. It might have been an idea to eat something the day before. The gap in my stomach jerked my head backwards when I tried to get sick again. I grabbed a few clumps of soggy toilet paper and tried to wipe the liquid from my mouth, from my cheeks, from my hands and from the cracks in between my fingers.

What I needed to set me right was a drink.

—Oh, Jesus.

First audible words of the day even though I don't believe in the man. No white in my eyes. Little red pin-pricks of spots just under my eyebrows. Come on, where the fuck are you, lad?

I remembered where I was when I got to the bar. But not how I got there. Still, a start is a start.

The joint was full of eager young stockbrokers eating their breakfast. And market traders drinking pints of Guinness. I was the only one wearing a tie and drinking a pint. I must have been at some do the night before.

The pint went down quick and left a scorch mark on my insides. A sign over the bar said that no one had ever managed to finish the pub's Special Mixed Grill. We had a chef like that one time in the King William and we had to get rid of her. Ha ha ha.

Nine o'clock. And still not a memory in the world about how I got where I was.

It was a grand warm morning. But I couldn't lift my head to look straight at the day. Too much fog. A foggy day in Paul Kelly's head. I felt like the postman in Rathbawn whose neck got damaged when a gate fell on him. His head hung to one side so he looked like he was sizing you up the whole time. The resulting thoughtful appearance got him picked on a lot of pub quiz teams.

The purposeful walk of people in the City. Aftershave and make-up everywhere. They kept brushing against me. I was way out of step. But keep going. Lift them and they'll fall themselves, my son. It was like an army walking over London Bridge. I seemed to be the only one going in the opposite direction. It made me feel like I was out in the wilds someplace. Looking at the Grand Canyon or some other such yoke that's supposed to humble you by its vastness.

I needed a cure. Past London Bridge station. Which was packed because the people who passed me on the bridge were the last in before the first IRA bomb scare of the day. Poor hoors stood on platforms all over Kent looking at their watches to see if they'd stopped.

I picked up one of those free magazines that always have features about eating out on docked boats and in Greek restaurants where they let you smash the plates. I flicked through it. Then I read every page while I waited for eleven. Opening time here.

Boogies' Wine Bar off Borough High Street looked just the job.

I knew if I had two more pints and went home I would feel well all day and not suffer till tomorrow morning. And that if I spent another day on the tear I wouldn't be able to drink tomorrow morning and by noon I'd be coming down so heavy the mad zone was a likely destination.

There were obvious advantages in hitting for home all right. But not just yet.

Boogies' Wine Bar was painted white and pink inside. It looked like Liberace's dream of the afterlife. A dozen men scattered around a horseshoe-shaped bar which had tropical fish swimming in tanks behind it. The barmaid was tall and blonde with a seam of savvy running through her face which made it difficult to look at even though she should have been attractive.

They'd been drinking for a while in Boogies' Wine Bar, judging by the uncollected glasses on the counter. Uncollected glasses. That really annoyed me. Banjaxed and all as I was.

3

So. I could have stood up Ms London and got a drink at ten o'clock. No. Probably not. How often did some poor gobshite walk in the wide-open door of the King William at nine o'clock in the morning and see twenty people on the last lap of an all-night lock-in only to hear the bad news.

—Sorry, mate, we're closed. Are you thick or something? Do you not know what the pub opening hours are?

Fairly often in fairness. Very often lately.

My mouth was filling up with water so I wobbled out towards the jacks. A star painted on the door. Like Miss Piggy's dressing-room in *The Muppet Show*.

It took me a few minutes to work out which jacks was which. The door of the men's had a sign, GIRLS, THIS WON'T DO.

The ladies' had BOYS, YOU CAN'T COME IN HERE.

I know I made the right choice because the jacks I picked had a row of cock-mangers along the wall. Still. You worry. All the time.

Me and Lydia were once going to put ELTON JOHN and OLIVIA NEWTON-JOHN signs on the toilet doors of the King William. But we didn't get around to it.

Most of the Boogies' faces were different when I came back to the bar. My pint was still left on the counter. It was flat and the head was down to a small scum over a few accusing bubbles.

Maybe the barmaid had left it there out of friendliness. She could have cleared it away. I smiled at her every time I ordered a fresh pint. She headed straight for the fruit machine when she broke at half-twelve. Tempus had fugited on me again.

I managed not to think of Lydia by the time I left Boogies'. The phone in the Tube station was working. Five rings. Vinnie answered. Perfectly.

—Hello, King William, how may I help you?

Vinnie. Professional and friendly to the last. His spake

deserved a question mark at the end because he did sound like he was wondering how he could help. Why wouldn't he be professional and friendly? I'd trained him well. He was nearly as good as me now. Only not quite. Not many people were. I heard the clinking of plates and the voice of Joan, the old dear who helped out in the kitchen sometimes.

—The special's lasagne, innit, love?

We sounded busy. That was good. Vinnie was asking me if I was OK. I realized I'd already come out with the line about being held up and I wouldn't be in for a couple of hours and I couldn't help it and would he be all right without me?

—I'd tell you if I was all right. If it was any of your business.

—Sorry, head. I was just wondering what to tell Kerrie.

—Tell her the usual. Say I'm at a meeting with the area manager or at a brewery conference or having lunch with Kennelly or anything. I'm sorry, so I am. Will you manage for the time being?

—The job is Oxo. Don't worry about it. There's plenty of us here.

—Hang about. Kerrie isn't supposed to be working today.

—She came in this morning to mind Kaya. Knocked the place up at nine. Said she had a feeling you wouldn't have got home. Boss, you haven't an idea of hell till you've heard Thomas the Tank Engine in a Kiwi accent before your breakfast.

—I'm sorry, Vinnie.

—It's all right. I'm recovering already. Have a couple more and get back here. Get back and get a few hours' kip in. Oh, shit, yeah, your Uncle Jimmy rang a couple of times this morning. Said it was urgent you give him a bell soon as poss. Wouldn't tell me anything, said it was family.

—Probably another oul grand-aunt kicking the bucket. The hoor can wait.

If I could have teleported directly back to the King William I would have. I did want to. I bought a travel card and got on the Northern Line. Two young bucks with a pit bull on the end of a steel chain sat across from me. One of them kept putting his face up against the dog's and rubbing noses with him. Then he'd land him a few clouts around the snot.

—Come on, you cunt. Come on, you wanker. Come on. You're my mate, intcha?

Some of the night before finally flickered through my mind. Just bits and pieces. Bits and pieces. Bits and pieces. Bits and pieces.

One of my old gaffers had bought his own pub in Stockwell. A free house. The Leprechaun. Formerly the Bricklayer's Arms. Mine hosts Patrick and Bridie O'Gara. It was the size of an Irish country church. Every manager in London was there. And all the bands. That was mainly what I remembered. Bits of songs. JCBs, Paddy and his bamboo, hearts in Ireland, sad fathers on Easter mornings and Sam Brown belts. Kennelly sang a Christy Moore song.

The compère was a tiny man with a gold watch on each wrist.

—And here's a request for a man here to sing an oul song for us. From just over the road in Brixton, Paul Kelly from the King William. Come on Paul and give us a few oul bars, you'll be singing soon enough anyways.

I was glad to get away from Kennelly and Hussey. Because I still wasn't pissed enough to miss the fact everyone I knew spoke to me in a semi-hush this weather. I tried to adjust the mike upwards so I wouldn't have to get down on my knees to sing into it.

—Go on, if there was hair on it, you'd manage it.

There was still only one song I could sing in tune.

6

You may travel far far from your own native home
Far away over the mountains, far away over the foam.
But of all the fine places that I've ever seen
Sure there's none to compare with the Cliffs of Dooneen.

Everyone knew the next bit.

I hit for Soho when I landed up west. Kennelly had once run a pub there where the barmaids wore schoolgirl outfits and every so often you'd see a middle-aged man washing his tie in the jacks bowl.

—Excuse me, sir.

—'Scuse me, love.

—Live bed show. Beautiful girls. Only two pounds.

Soho was full of angry middle-aged men shooting out of doorways. Steaming with anger in the heat. The puzzled anger kids have when someone's clobbering them on the back of the head and they can't work out who it is. The men went into those doorways furtive and looked over their shoulders. And they came out of them angry and looked straight ahead at nothing. Cars narrowly missed them as they crossed the streets.

Me and Lydia walked through Soho one night. We walked through it plenty of nights, what am I on about? But perhaps this was our first night out together. We had a meal in Leicester Square. Planet Spaghetti or something like that. I ordered lasagne because already I knew this was special enough for me not to make a fool of myself eating pasta in front of her. Lydia whirled spaghetti bolognaise into her mouth as effortlessly as if it was on a conveyor belt. The *Generation Game* conveyor belt because she never gave any impression of haste.

We saw a film in the Odeon that night as well. *Wall Street*, I think. She bought me a pair of red braces for my birthday which was the week after. But I'm not sure it was *Wall Street* because drink dumps all memories into one teeming stew

7

like the Lancashire hotpot which appears on the lunch menu of the King William in four differently monickered guises every week.

I'm sure this was a rainy night and we had no umbrella. Still we stopped to watch a young man and woman with short haircuts pace up and down in front of a Continental-style brasserie. Self-styled. The man shouting in a Sarf London accent.

—You think that nobody cares for you, don't you? All of you think that. But someone does. He does. But do you know his name? Jesus Christ, that's his name. He cares for you, for all of you. But you've got to listen to his word. To his word. You have to fall on your knees and say, 'Lord I am a sinner. Lord, I am full of sin and filth and evil but I can change. I can change and I will change and listen to your word.'

—Oh, fuck.

Lydia shook rain droplets out of her hair.

—It's Gary God.

—I'd think of him more as Trevor Christ.

A couple of winos gathered around the preacher. One of them danced in front of him and shouted:

—Hallelujah.

The other stood beside him and looked like he'd found an escaped zoo animal. He circled the preacher and blew gently into his ear. Two men in black leather jackets and Levi 501s walked over and shoved the two interlopers out of the way. They hit the dancing wino across the head when he refused to move.

—God needs bouncers.

I whispered it to Lydia. I thought it was too good a line to only use once, so I said it to the small man beside me with the neatly trimmed beard.

—Look. God needs bouncers.

He didn't seem to hear me, so I pumped up the volume.

—Look. God needs bouncers.

Most of the spit that jumped out of his mouth landed in his beard.

—The servants of the Lord need protection because of those evil and ignorant people who would stop them doing their work. The day is at hand when Armageddon will be visited upon the Earth and there will be a great wailing and gnashing of teeth. The unbelievers will all be cast into the pit and suffer great torment for ever. Think of it, friend. You know where you will be.

I thought it was very funny. Lydia didn't. She talked about it for weeks. She said she got a shiver every time she thought of the man with the neatly trimmed beard.

Maybe it had meant something. You get to the stage where you don't laugh at anything. Because everything is equally funny.

A woman with a henna pony-tail played 'Merrily Kissed the Quaker' on a mandolin in Oxford Circus Tube. It was three o'clock, so there was plenty of room in the carriages. The Victoria Line would take me home. I would be back in the pub by four o'clock. I would have a bath and my heart might slow down for a few minutes so I could get a couple of hours' kip and then there wouldn't be that much left in the day.

I got off at Brixton Tube and walked under the railway bridge.

—We're backing Brixton.

Soca music blared from the take-away that sold curried goat and kept getting busted for dope. It was four o'clock. I could be in the pub by ten past four. It would be quiet. I walked up and down in front of the Crown and Castle for a couple of minutes before I ducked in.

I didn't head back to the King William after the first one. Or after the next one. It didn't matter a continental fuck whether we were busy or not. It was a day when I couldn't face the people. Not yet. Vinnie would look after everything and consider it a miracle when I finally got back. I was nicely cut again anyhow. That was a relief.

Someone stuck on a few songs to stain the silence. One of them about this sketch who drinks loads and dies and then everyone is really sorry for him. Gas. There I was listening to this and feeling sorry for me.

Jukeboxes. It's what they're there for. To give people a soundtrack for the film they've cast themselves in. The second worst thing about being on the batter is constructing these masterpieces with the TobySoundtrack. And the worst is knowing you're doing it and wondering what the people who love you would think if they saw you.

My daughter Kaya. My dead wife Lydia. My young brother Johnny. I'd be all right if he was here. You need someone you can depend on. He should have landed over to England. Fuck him. No. What did Mam always say about me and Johnny?

—There's a pair of ye in it.

The best I could think of at that moment was the start of the night before. The memory of us in the public bar of the King William before we hit off for the Captain Christy. Kennelly, Hussey, myself, and Kerrie beside me. She broke away occasionally to look at Kaya's new doll. They'd bought it in a Camden shop that sold God's amount of yokes from the arse-end of South America. I remembered Kerrie saying it came from Venezuela.

—Veyenizwella.

There can't be many worse words for someone from New Zealand to say.

—Nuh Zilland.

The first pint. Three pints in about an hour and a half. Even Vinnie smiling as he planked them down on the bar. Talk and jokes and the right memories. My steady voice.

—Jesus, I feel brilliant. I'll take it easy enough tonight. I want to feel this good tomorrow.

Maybe believing it. And maybe other people believing it too. I couldn't drag back the memory of the end of the night though. It squirted away from me the way a football does when your sleeping dream puts you in the number nine jersey for Ireland in a World Cup final.

The door of the public bar of the King William creaked when I flung it open. There was football on the telly but I didn't look up at it. I was climbing the stairs up to the living quarters when I heard Vinnie calling me. Like I expected. I should have kept walking.

—Paul, where the fuck were you? Come on, I was expecting you back by the afternoon. And you're fucking langered.

—I'm all right. Do you know I didn't have that much . . .

—Fuck's sake. If bullshit was music, you'd be a brass band.

—I'm OK. I can hold my drink.

—Ah, what's the fucking point?

—Look, Sonny Jim, I'm still the fucking boss, right? Nothing big went wrong did it? I said I'm sorry, didn't I?

—You didn't, you know.

—I did.

—It's nothing to do with the pub. Look, Kerrie is here all day. She's worried sick about you. I told her you were like a bad oul mongrel and you'd come home in the end but she's been crying and everything, like.

—Muttley. That's me. Muttley Kelly and his dastardly dick.

—It's not funny. See, I told you you were elephants. And Kaya. Kaya is worrying all day and asking where her daddy is. Jesus, I even went up and looked after her for an hour so Kerrie could get a bite to eat. Come on, Paul, you do give a shite about Kaya? Fuck the pub but your . . .

—Yeah, yeah, yeah. Fuck the pub. I'm sorry, that's twice I've said it. Where are they?

—In your bedroom. Oh, and your uncle rang again. Uncle Jimmy. Ring him pronto, he says.

—Let him wait. Cheers, mate.

I went to the bathroom before I braved the bedroom. My eyes were burrowing back into my head. I wiped under them with a tissue. The skin there looked damp and black but the tissue was dry and white when I took it away.

Kerrie was braiding Kaya's hair into corn-row. They didn't even look back at me when I walked in. I clapped my hands over Kerrie's eyes.

—Boo, it's the monster.

—Ahhh, ahhh.

—Dad, look at my hair. Kerrie says it's called corn-row.

—You shit, Paul, I didn't even hear you come in.

—Be alert. The world needs more lerts. Your hair is lovely, pet. I had to meet Mr O'Neill today, that was why I wasn't here.

—Me and Kerrie had a nice day, Dad. We went to the park and fed the squirrels and then the Alsatians came along and chased them up the trees but they couldn't catch any of them.

—Alsatians are very silly, Kaya. They used be called German —

—She wants to tell you about her day, Paul.

Kerrie's insistent Kiwi vowels. They could lay down the law to anyone. If she'd had the ounce of inclination she didn't seem to own.

—And we went to McDonald's. And I had fries and a milk shake and we were going to go to the market but Kerrie said we had to come back here because you would be here and you'd wonder where we were gone.

Kerrie reminded me Uncle Jimmy had been ringing all day. I should ring him, bad and all as he was.

Kaya had fallen asleep like a tiny version of her mother. Motionless. The lads in the public bar used keep going on about how she was the dead-down spit of Lydia. Now they said nothing about that although Del still sometimes plucked fifty-pence pieces from behind her ears.

The phone beside the bed rang. I bellied up towards it. Vinnie's voice. Calm Vinnie. The cool, clean hero.

—It's your uncle again. Do you feel up to talking to him?

—Oh, go ahead. Or he'll bankrupt himself with these fucking phone calls. If he's not calling reverse.

—Hello.

—Hello.

—Hello.

—Hello, Jimmy, spit it out, what's up with you? Did you win the Lotto or do you want me to ring you back?

—Oh, Jesus, Paul, thank the Lord I've got hold of you.

—That's very nice of you. What's the story?

—Oh, Jesus, Paul, oh, Jesus. Your mother kept saying to ring you. She's under sedation now. She was in an awful panic.

—It's not her nerves acting up again, is it?

—It's Johnny. He's dead. He was dead when they got him to the hospital.

—Johnny?

—Johnny. Johnny your brother. This morning. He was attacked coming home from the pub. Someone bet the head off him.

—Ah, now, fucking hold on here.

—He's dead.

—Johnny.

Johnny twirled in my head, clicking his thumbs in the air while he danced with two girls from Courtney's Travel Agents at the same time.

—The cops say they have a clue who done it. Jesus, he was rightly bursted.

—Who?

—Johnny.

He kept twirling. The blue and black flecks flew strange colours on to the floor as they collided with the Spiders' disco lights. Somewhere I heard him laugh and tell me things were grand.

—Who fucking done it?

—I haven't a notion. I'm ringing from yere house.

The feeling inside my head was like the colour red. The real unmixed one. I wanted to punch someone.

—That'd fucking figure.

—Your mammy is in a bad way but most of the neighbours are here. What did you say before that?

—Nothing. Nothing for you to bother your pretty little head about.

—Don't take that cheeky tone with me. I'm killing myself all day trying to get hold of you.

—But you're still alive.

And Johnny was dead. Someone had killed him. Out of spite. So I'd never hear him call my name again. The old thoughts came back. A buzzing plane flying across a broken pool of sky and the word 'revenge' came up in a smoke trail.

—The funeral is on Friday. To give you and a few others a chance to get back.

—I might be busy. Jimmy, what happened?

—You can't be that busy. Just because you're doing well beyond. And we're all proud of you. You have to come back, you know you have to. Do you give a shite about your family at all, do you?

—Yeah. I suppose so.

I hung up. Kerrie was gone to the Greek for some nosh. I suddenly copped how drunk I was. And maybe had been for a while. I heard Jimmy again telling me Johnny was dead but I only sort of heard it too. Like it was behind a screen. Or on TV. Poor old Roy Castle, wasn't it tough on him all the same and used he be deadly on *The Record Breakers*?

My brother Johnny wasn't my brother Johnny now. He didn't exist any more. That was it. From this morning Johnny hadn't ever been born. No one would ever have to think of him again when they were arranging anything.

His face. I tried to assemble it in my mind. Shivering. Because I wasn't sure if I had it exactly right. And the memory could only get worse from now on. And it would be a different face after eight years anyways.

Jimmy knew the story about me and home. He knew I was out of all that. Like the reformed villains in the Seventies films who couldn't even be tempted back by Mr Big for one last job.

—One last job, just one last job, bubba, then you're out of the rackets for good.

I never went back. No, I never went back. Not once. I turned down all those plates of turkey and ham with my name on them at the connected communions and confirmations and twenty-firsts and weddings and funerals. I made my excuses and never left for home. Home to me was where I lived. I was never drunk enough to want to go back to Rathbawn.

Love never brought me back. Hate would now.

Kerrie walked into the bedroom. She held two patterned plates with lamb kebabs on them. The strands of purple cabbage dangled over the edge of mine.

—Eat this, you'll feel better in no time. There's some nice white wine in the fridge if you're up to it or red if you'd prefer it.

Johnny was a ghost. He had always been one. Because of this morning. I'd picked a ghost to play on the same team as me on the pitch with the crooked tubular steel goalposts behind Rathbawn Dispensary. He used wear an identical strip to mine. A blue Puma jersey that was far too warm and too big for him. But nothing would do him only to get it.

—Are you the best footballer in Ireland?

A question he'd always ask as we made painfully slow progress up the hill towards the Dispensary because his cogs were sliding and slewing off the tarmac. He wore them over from home because he couldn't manage to tie the laces on his boots yet and he wouldn't let me do it for him in front of the other lads. The faint mix of sentiment and jealousy I felt when he played well seemed to be repeating on me.

The coughing and spluttering I could almost hear again. Waking Mam up to look for the nebulizer in the night. An hour then. Tops. Semi-silence. And more coughs. He was on the verge of the Rovers team. I could see him homing in on goal and then the spin away with the hand in the air as a smile graced those teeth chipped when he fell down the stairs that time. When he was five. He would always spin away now. For ever.

Ah, no, not fucking tears above all things. For who these tears? For him? For me? Maybe for him and me and something else?

—My brother's dead. Someone killed him last night.

Kerrie's finger pushed rice methodically on to her fork. Shocking Pink nail varnish. The tears rolled down my face. Snots and clots in my eyes and nose.

—I'm cracking. My brother is after dying and I'm really cracking up. I'm gone, gone.

—Oh, shit, Paul, I didn't know. Were you close?

—I don't know. I don't have a fucking clue.

—I'll put the food in the oven. You can eat it later.

—I'm cracking, Kerrie. I can't take any more of this. It's not on.

—You're not cracking. Come on, look, if you were really going crazy you wouldn't know you were.

—Oh, great, I'm fucking ultra-sane then.

—Maybe you are.

—Tell Vinnie. Please tell Vinnie. I want Vinnie to know.

—What was your brother's name.

—Johnny. John. Johnny really. Tell Vinnie.

I rested my head against her bony hip that wasn't quite right in some way and made her walk with legs bent outwards so she looked about to perform an act of contortion. Some days it looked well. She moved like jelly. I breathed in the odour of hip and flesh and sweat. It smelt like something alive.

—I'll tell Vinnie. I'll stay tonight, Paul.

—Please. Leave the food. I'll eat it. It's still middlin' warm.

I horsed through the kebabs. The cold rice seemed suitable. Eleven o'clock. Vinnie's voice. Like I expected. Again.

—Boss, you all right?

—Sound, Vinnie. I'll be down in a bit. I'm just on the blower.

Missus Jordan answered the phone at Mam's house. Or Missus Doran. I wasn't sure of the voice. I just left the message that I'd be home for the funeral and hung up before they could ask any questions.

I went to the wardrobe. Five past. I hadn't worn my best suit since the night myself and Lydia had our official baptism as head honchos of this pub. I locked the bedroom door and fucked my clothes into a heap on the floor.

A look at my body in the mirror. Body was right. Healthier corpses over in King's College Hospital with tags on their toes reading 'Death by misadventure'. The belly swollen by all these months of porter. A couple of grey lumps around the hip left over from the psoriasis I had when I was a nipper. Red marks on the side of the hips where the thirty-four waist was splaying out to a thirty-six. And, Jesus, the knees were gone as bandy.

The clothes went into a bag. When they made that bag it stayed made. Colmcille United U-15, League and Cup champions 1982–83. And hardly a mark on it. Kerrie rapped the door.

—Paul, are you OK? Can I come in?

—Down in a sec, Kel. Could you ask Vinnie to make a few sandwiches. Give him a hand. Tell him to ring the nick and all and say we're having a small private party here after hours.

—Are you sure? Are you OK?

—Yeah. Go on. I'll be down in a mo. Go on. I swear I'm OK.

On with the Betty Boop boxer shorts and a pair of blue socks. Grandad Kelly was so banjaxed with arthritis he had a twelve-inch square of plastic to help him get his socks on. He had a shoe-horn as well. I squatted and rubbed Punch Quick-Shine across my boat shoes after I threw on my trousers. At least a hundred applications. I kind of heard Lydia's voice when I flung my jacket on over a white shirt. I shrugged my shoulders so the jacket hung properly. The voice would have come from back on the bed. She would have been easing on a pair of tights.

—You know, you can look really well when you make the effort. Not many people are able to wear a suit properly.

I nearly had the bedroom door unlocked when I remembered and went back to the wardrobe. Ties. Burnt brown, dark purple, dark pink, dark green all together. Green-and-red paisleys, red, blue and light-green triangles, light-red and yellow circles on dark red. Red with light-blue octagons.

Lydia would buy ties when we had a serious barney. She bought me six in three years. Then she stopped. I could hear Vinnie foghorning people out of the pub.

The bar was half empty when I got down. Except tonight it was half full. Maybe. Vinnie and Sligo Mick and Jo from Portsmouth were almost pouring the gargle down people's throats and moving them into the street by force. Kerrie ground her feet into the carpet. Wondering if she should bring out the sandwiches yet. I kissed her on the back of the neck and filled two glasses of Liebfraumilch from the optic.

—C'mere.

I opened the door of the little kitchen where we bred the hotpot. We heard the jukebox being plugged out and a few muffled groans of protest from the art college students who didn't really care because there was a warehouse party on just over the road.

The kitchen light danced, shimmered and went out. I kicked the door outwards so we could see each other. All the dishes had been cleared away. The stubs of Joan's Gold Flakes were placed neatly side by side in the plastic Bulmers ashtray.

—Cheers.

—Cheers.

Clink. Off-centredly.

—*Merci, garçon.*

—Jesus, this stuff is foul piss.

—Aw, Paul, don't spoil the moment.

I slipped out to the bar to fill two more glasses. Vinnie had the place nearly cleared. The regulars sat at the bar.

—Kerrie, you know I'll have to go back to the funeral.

—I know. You'll have to go soon, yeah?

—Tomorrow morning. I'm bringing Kaya with me.

—It's going to be awful for you, isn't it?

—You see, Kel, the brewery owe me a lot of time. I might spend a couple of weeks back in Ireland. There might be some things need straightening out.

—I understand that. You've got to go home. He was your brother.

—But it's just I think it would be better if I went back to Ireland on my own. I just think it would be better, like.

—It's all right. I wouldn't expect you to bring me.

And that made me sadder than I ever had been when I looked at her. Because she should have expected it. She had a right to after all.

—It's AOK, Paul. Just one thing though.

—Which?

—I don't expect you to come back.

—Now you're being shagging silly. Come on, before these bastards have all the sambos devoured.

Vinnie hoisted the sandwiches on to the counter when we came out of the kitchen. Then he remoted the television back on and powerboats plunged effortlessly across an obscure stretch of Swiss lake. I started pulling pints of lager.

—These are on me, lads. I'll be away for a while so make the most of it. Vinnie's from Cavan so ye know what to expect.

Except most of them didn't because they'd never been to Ireland. Del eased his Greenpeace-friendly bulk off his stool. The rest of the regulars theatrically withdrew from their pints and rested their hands on their knees.

—Paul, I'd just like to say how sorry we are. Vinnie told us about your trouble and on behalf of all the punters and members of the Committee we'd just like to offer our support. We hope you enjoy your time back in Eire. We can't think of anyone deserves a break more than you do.

The Committee launched into a round of applause and Del sat down.

—Vinnie, rig up the video and stick in the football tapes.

We watched King William United make their jerky camcordered way across the mudflats of Sydenham, Norwood, Blackheath and Streatham.

—Forward wind that. We got beat seven–nil in that one. It was the day after Wayne's stag.

Laughter at Vinnie trying a spectacular overhead kick and falling flat on his back into a heap of muck by the penalty spot. Then the camcorder panned to Lydia and Del's wife in a fit of the giggles under a huge Heineken umbrella. Lydia gave a thumbs-up. I caught Del's eye. I didn't need to look at anyone else.

The punters all left together at half two, venturing into the Brixton night and singing. Del wanted to know where I was going in the morning. I hadn't thought of that. I said Euston. Flying gave me the willies. I turned down a slew of lift offers and told them I'd be away for two weeks at the most. Del embraced me as I opened the door to let them out.

—I just want to let you know that whatever's happened and all that, we all still think you're a good geezer.

A tapping on the window at five o'clock. The Jamaican woman who painted herself white so she'd look like an angel. Every time they brought her back to the hospital they cleaned it off. The brilliance of the new paint on her face showed she'd escaped that morning. She moved off for Coldharbour Lane and hummed a Lovers' Rock hit to herself.

—She frightens the shit out of me.

—She's harmless. Before she got really bad, she used come in here early in the day and buy fags and crisps. She had lovely manners.

—You won't come back.

Kerrie's voice surprised us. She hadn't said anything since we opened the second bottle of Southern Comfort. Just buried her head in the crook of her arm and leaned against the Give Us a Break quiz machine beside her chair. I walked her up the stairs and asked her if she trusted me.

Asleep, she liked to hoist her right leg into the air and clamp it around me. Sometimes she squeezed so hard my leg went dead. I lay awake with sweat creeping and crawling down my chest and across my hips and tried to pick out shapes in the dark by looking straight into it.

I wanted to make sense of Kerrie's sleeping breaths too. They sounded like

—I-you, I-you, I-you, I-you, I-you.

The dream came to me again that night. The same one from all these nights I fell asleep with that clinging clay thirst in my mouth.

I am young and I am walking along this country road wearing a stripy T-shirt and a pair of shorts. It is a dry, dusty road surrounded by fields of green grass. There's a heat haze coming up off the road and I feel my tongue swelling up and hurting me because it is so dry.

I come across a pump. One of those old blue parish pumps. I pull the handle and water flows out of it. The water is silver like brand-new ten-pence coins and sparkling in the sun like on ads and it is the most refreshing drink I've ever had.

Every moment of the dream is with me when I wake up. But what annoys me is not knowing where it comes from. They had those pumps out the country one time. But I never saw one in Rathbawn. And I never drank from one.

Two

A Father to Millions

Morning woke Matthew by poking a golden finger of sunlight into his eyes. That was the first line of a book I took out of the National School library one time. I can't remember anything else about it except it might have been one where you scratched the page and a faint smell of lilac air-freshener was released.

Morning. And what a lovely morning. My head felt like it had been used as the ball in the United match the night before. I eased my leg away from Kerrie.

Half-eight. The red Teasmade digits winked at me. Eight thirty-one. Kerrie stayed asleep. Zonked. Not used to it. Still not used to me. After nearly two years.

I still felt a bit drunk. That looking-at-your-life-on-MTV feeling. Dazed and confused. I tiptoed down

23

to the bar and rang Euston. Next train to Holyhead eleven o'clock. Sound job.

Holyhead four. Ferry out six. Dublin ten. Stay some place. Train down at one. Rathbawn three. Rathbawn town of high renown. What was the rhyme the boggers used have?

> Rathbawn, town of high renown,
> And church without a steeple.
> In every door
> There stands a whore
> To laugh at decent people.

A day and a bit before I'd see good old Rathbawn town. For the first time in eight years. Eight years since.

—Your honour, my client has given me an undertaking that he will seek work in England. He has hopes of gaining employment there. This is a first offence.

—Does he realize the seriousness of this, Mr Flynn? I don't want him to think he can escape the consequences of his actions just by leaving the country.

—Oh, he's very contrite, your honour. This is completely out of character for him.

—Well then, perhaps. But I don't want him to skulk back into the jurisdiction within a couple of weeks.

I wouldn't mind but it was a silly row over nothing. I hadn't raised a hand to anyone since. The guy didn't eat anything except soup for a couple of months after. He was five years older than me. Going on for the guards. Lack of respect for my betters. The old problem.

Vinnie stumbled around upstairs in blue underpants and a T-shirt. He was white in the face. All I got from Malta was this lousy T-shirt.

—Lousy T-shirt, hey, sir, lousy T-shirt, you want lousy T-shirt?

—I'll tell O'Neill you're taking holidays after the funeral. There won't be any hass.

Kaya was so still when she slept. Don't sleep like that because you remind me of the dead. Poem from school. The shape of Lydia's bones in her face. The cut of her smig.

—Kaya, wake up, come on, rise and shine, the clock's struck nine.

I helped her dress. She was getting more independent the whole time. Pre-school. Great idea. Loads of friends. She got up early for it. Anxious to be out there in the world. Let's go to work.

But she was tired this morning. I knew by the serious face she put on. Don't mess with the best 'cause the best don't mess. She narrowed the eyebrows and pushed out the top lip. Investing every movement with ponderous significance. Like a method actor on a bad day. Brushing her teeth. Sorting out the hair. Looking at the reflection from both sides. Tilting the head to the left. Then to the right. Vain for four. Bright for it too.

—What d'you think?

—Simply the best, Kaya, better than all the rest.

—What'll I wear, Dad?

—Your best clobber.

—My best clobber, yeah.

Giggles. Del talking to her one evening in the bar.

—You got your best clobber on, Kaya. What you got on? Your best clobber.

I poured out the Coco Pops. Her favourite cereal. Jesus, the sacrifices you make for your kids. Me with this stomach on me having to look at that brown scum on top of the milk. I put marmalade and butter on two slices of toast for her. She was beginning to make me nervous. This dread that one day she would find me boring.

—We're going on a big journey today.

She wasn't listening. Fuck me, I didn't know they still put plastic dinosaurs in cereal packets.

—Kaya, listen to me like a good *cailín*.

—Sorry, Dad.

—It's OK. We're going on a big journey today so we're going to pack some of your clothes and toys and things.

—Where we going?

Just like that. Down to business.

—We're going to Ireland. Back to where I was born. Where Granny Kelly is from. We're going to go on a train and then across the seven seas on a boat. You'll see where I come from.

—Ireland, mmmm.

—You'll like it. We'll just be there for a short while.

—I'd like to see Granny Kelly. Is she older than Granny Calder?

Lydia's mum came down a few months ago to see us. Her husband didn't. I couldn't blame him. He didn't blame me.

—Will we see Grandad Kelly?

—No, he's not at home.

—Is he with Mum in heaven?

—No, he's not. But Mum is in heaven all right.

You tell yourself you'll never say these sorts of things but then you feel you owe it to the kid.

—I wish I could see my grandads.

—You'll see your granny. You can show her how well you can read and how big you've grown. She'll make a big fuss out of you. You'll be the pet.

—I'm not a pet.

—All right. You're not.

When I was growing up in the Park all I seemed to have were relations. If some lad threw a stone at me or some girl kicked a football back to me, Mam would tell me we were related some way. Colmcille Park. Kaya couldn't even remember her own mother. Mam wrote to her sometimes. Birthday cards. Christmas.

—I'd love to see you.

Mam knew how I felt about home. She still wrote to Kaya.

—I'd love to see you, your Granny Kelly.

Kaya sent drawings back. Bits she'd done on paper. Bits she'd done out of colouring books. She had some patience. Finishing whole colouring books in a day. I don't think I ever finished a picture.

Vinnie was eating a sandwich downstairs at the counter. The clock over his head said ten. For one second the slouch of his shoulders reminded me of Johnny.

—Vinnie, call me a cab, will you.

—Go on, Kaya, you say it to him.

—Dad, you're a cab.

I was like a poisoned pup I was. I often thought of taking up smoking so a fag in the morning might do something for me. I hit down to the bar. Vinnie was calling. The cab firm were great. Always on the spot on the dot.

Errol landed in. Rasta Man Errol. Always in the Soul Food take-away at night. Someone told me he owned it. Kaya was much livelier now. Probably thinking of all the boasting she'd do about her trip when she came back. She loved telling stories. She was class at it. Timing, punchlines, she had the full monty.

—'Bye, Kaya, look after the oul guy.

—'Bye, Vinnie, this time next year we'll both be millionaires.

Told you she was bright for four. She picks up phrases like that off the television and uses them correctly. The latest favourite was:

—Do not disturb my scientific work.

This was out of a film with dragons and princesses and swordfighting and so on in it. It wasn't a half-bad flick.

—I'll give you a shout during the week, Vinnie, see how things are getting on.

—Don't even think of it.

Kaya looked out the window of the cab. A little wet circle appeared where her nose rubbed against it. Rapt I think is the word. Her eyes flicked and fluttered in as many directions as she could manage at the one time.

Errol amber-gambled twice for us. His skin was black black. *Noir*. It looked deeper than mine. Prince Far I was on the stereo. Chanting about flying.

—Good song, this one.

Prince Far I. He got murdered. Like Johnny. Prince Far I would have been a hardy sketch. His friends wouldn't have let it go. You can't let people destroy the things you love. Once maybe but not twice.

I wonder would the family have come over to visit me if I hadn't said I wanted nothing to do with home. Addresses never sent. Until the letter I sent Mam after Lydia. After Lydia. But I stayed cut off. Like the oul lad. Terse Christmas-card exchanges. Sheep pitter-patting their way through snow to Rathbawn with the shepherds behind them. Travelling from Harlesden, from Norwood, from Peckham, from Brixton. Just once back and I might know what Johnny looked like. It wouldn't have killed me.

—You going to need a hand with them bags.

—Ah, no, it's all right. No hass. I'll get them up some way.

—You going to need a hand. You can't manage them. You got to carry the little lady. She not going to walk up all them steps, is she?

The steps up at Euston. Fucksakes. Who did they build them for? Mr Memory. As punishment. You'll remember steps the next time, you fat fuck.

—Kaya, piggybacks.

—Shoulderbacks.

—Come off it, don't waste time. Shoulderbacks is too dangerous.

—Shoulderbacks, Dad.

—Shoulderbacks it is then.

Errol shook hands with me when we reached the summit. He did the same with Kaya but with more respect.

—You behave yourself, you hear, Kaya, you got a proud name.

—All right, Errol.

—Have a nice trip, mate. And look after the little lady. A man can be a father to millions but he can be a dad to only a few.

Errol said things like that all the time. In a voice of extreme seriousness. Like he was auditioning for the part of Malcolm X. He loped down the steps.

The Irish Mail. All those hours and then the fucking crossing. Still, on the plane you could be there and then you wouldn't be there. Like Air India. Bang. You'd never know anything. The same could happen on the boat. The *Estonia*. But I always feel I'd have the opportunity to swim to safety. Some control over my fate. Control. Important to cod yourself it exists.

We played Snap as the train pulled away from London. And Happy Families. Neither of us knew the rules but we played because we liked the pictures on the cards. Kaya was asleep when we got to Crewe. A bubble bobbed around the surface of my stomach so I drank a couple of cans of the Löwenbräu I had packed.

She woke when we got to Holyhead. Eight years ago I'd been there with a hundred quid in my pocket and three addresses in London that all proved to be wrong. I wouldn't even be able to talk to that me now. You become so different from yourself sometimes it seems a waste of time to have lived that life at all.

—Get the fuck out of here, Dad, said Kaya as I left her down at the top of the gangway.

Maybe I should have chided her but there's worse things going on than cursing, isn't there? We sat in the Comfort Lounge as the ferry hauled its way out of Holyhead and towards the past. A different country, as the man says.

We should have crossed at night. I couldn't think of what to do with Kaya for the four hours so I made her put her coat on. I reckoned it might get chilly in the evening.

—I'm bored, Dad.

—D'you want to go to sleep?

—I can't sleep because it's not night.

—You'll be tired later.

—But I'm not tired now.

I didn't get much comfort from the Comfort Lounge. I woke Kaya and brought her to the main bar with me. The Guinness was foul. My companion had no complaints about the Coke. She bubbled out a laugh when the sea sent her glass sliding down the table. I caught it. She kept an eye on it for a few minutes. I nudged it a couple of times with the side of my hand when I thought her attention was wavering.

—Want a game of Snakes and Ladders, Dad?

—Sure thing.

Anything except fucking Ludo.

It was a long game. I won it. And the second. Every time Kaya came near the end in the third game she hit a snake. I noticed her biting her lip when a five brought her to the gormless-looking serpent who ran from ninety-four to twenty-seven. I rushed her counter six spaces forward. She looked at me quickly. Blank gaze back. Another five for Kaya. Victory.

Three more hours of Snakes and Ladders to go. And I didn't win another game. The drink sped up some of the hours and minutes in the dark but not them all.

The big houses in Howth had a good look down at us as

we got near to the North Wall. Kaya tried to be interested when I told her about Ireland's Eye and Lambay and Vikings but she was getting drowsy.

—This is Ireland, Kaya. Home sweet home.

—Oh. We staying in Granny Kelly's tonight then?

—No. We'll stay in a hotel. You'll see Granny Kelly tomorrow. You need a good night's sleep, kiddo.

—Mmmm.

My daughter's first sight of Ireland was the dirt of the ferry terminal. Even the walls of the building looked tired. It hadn't changed much. The word home was skipping in and out of my mind. I tried to stop it but I couldn't. I was being dragged back. It had started. Kaya sucked her thumb as we escorted our bags down the ramp from the boat.

A taxi man dropped us off at a hotel on the quays. I never thought I would have to stay in a hotel in Dublin. Or that I would be able to. The woman at reception smiled down at Kaya when we booked in and didn't pay me much heed.

—Your hair is lovely. What's your name?

—Kaya, K-A-Y-A.

—That's an unusual name. What does it mean?

—A song. It's a song, it is.

The receptionist told me I had a lovely daughter and the residents' bar stayed open all night. Her jaw dropped when she heard Kaya's accent after my lovely Midland brogue. Attractive, sonorous, rugged. Rathbawn.

I hadn't even thought of it before. That Kaya had an English accent. A Sarf London accent. Fink. Fings. 'Aven't. Awright. Wossaten, Dad? She was my kid but she didn't sound anything like me. Or her mother. Or Granny Kelly or any of my relations. Eight years ago the only people I'd heard speaking in that accent were on *Minder*. Funny that your kid can grow up foreign.

Dropping off to sleep, I realized I wanted to talk to Kerrie.

For once it was something I wanted to do. I thought I could phone straight out to England but I was wrong and had a puzzled exchange with someone at reception before I hung up.

Who killed my brother? The thought woke me up for a few minutes at four o'clock. The sweat squelched under me as I pivoted before going asleep again.

Back awake at six o'clock. As well off getting the nine train. Another cab. At Connolly Station I decided to ring Mam and tell her we were on our way. She never slept more than a couple of hours a night so I knew she'd be up. Washing dishes, emptying ashes and setting fires even though she was home alone now. I could see her kneeling over the fireplace with the blue housecoat just covering her knees, rolling up thin pieces of newspaper, and I would have cancelled the call if she hadn't picked the receiver up on the second bleep.

—Hello . . . hello.

She sounded like she expected the caller to start giving her dog's abuse.

—Hello.

—Hello. Who's that? Who is that?

—Hello, Mam, it's me, Paul.

—Oh, Jesus, Paul, where are you?

—Connolly, going getting the train down, I'll be there in a few hours.

—Oh, that's great. Is there anyone with you?

—Kaya, your granddaughter. Do you want to speak to her? We don't have a lot of money left.

—Paul, are you sure you're OK for money? Will you be all right?

—I'm rolling in money, Mam. I just have fuck-all change for the phone.

—Don't shout at me.

—I'm not shouting at you.

—It's just my nerves haven't been good these last few days. I always warned ye not to get involved in rows, didn't I? Poor Johnny, and him doing so well for himself lately.

—I'm sorry, Mam. Do they know who did it?

—No. No one knows. Everyone has been awful nice to me.

—Mam. Kaya wants to talk to you.

—Hello, Granny, hiya.

—. . .

—Yes, Dad says we'll be down soon.

—. . .

—Thanks for all the presents, Granny Kelly.

—. . .

—I am being a good girl, Dad says I am.

—. . .

—'Bye.

Kaya handed me the receiver.

—You'll be down this afternoon, Paul.

—I'll be down around eleven. See you then. I'm out of change.

—Be sure and mind yourself.

Two fifty-pence pieces rattled accusingly against the bottom of the call-box when I hung up.

—Here, Kaya, we'll buy chocolate with these. The machine gave them back to us, isn't that great?

The old home town still looked the same when you stepped down from the train. Who were the two mean and mysterious strangers, and what had brought them out West to Bord Na Mona Gulch? It was Quick-Draw Kelly and Kaya the Kid.

Quick-Draw's trigger-finger was itchy. But first. Kaya paused from scraping a splintering twig against the walls of the shops we trudged past.

—I'm hungry, Dad.

Good thinking, Kaya the Kid.

—Right, I'll get you crisps in . . . this place . . . here.

Next door to Neary's Newsagents was a pub with some dirty Rathbawn Rovers flags drooping out of a smoky grey upstairs window. The Sportsman's Bar? Where the fuck had that come out of? Eight years is a long time but. But not as long as twenty-one years. Which is a mighty long time.

—We'll go in here and I'll get you a bottle of Fanta as well.

—Get what?

—A bottle of orange.

Fanta. I hadn't said that in years. Remember if you say lemonade here you get the red stuff.

—White lemonade, mate, what other sort is there?

Half, not a glass. Bitter, not beer.

No one behind the counter. No brewery inspectors down this neck of the woods checking the quality of service. Red leather couches along the side walls. Like a steak house that filled up with Geordies at the weekend. Where was this fucking barman?

He strolled in from the jacks. A smell of disinfectant crystals off his hands. He wiped them with an involuntarily multi-hued dishcloth lying on the counter. Slow wipe. I'm not killing myself to get you a drink. Don't worry, son, I'm not dying for one. Yet. Drawl.

—Pint of Guinness, sham. Bottle of orange and a couple of packs of crisps. And a straw for the orange.

—Can I have two straws, Dad?

—Sorry, sham, could you give us four straws?

I wish I could do some exciting trick with straws to impress my daughter. Or is it with balloons you do it? You can do it with straws as well though.

Two women with prams came in the door. One of them had a little boy walking along with her as well. Around

Kaya's age. I was the oldest person in the pub. The pair of women were hardly twenty. One of them exchanged a cursory kiss with the barman. Like the nose-rub of an Eskimo in bad form.

Kaya and the new boy in town looked at each other. Hello. Hello. They ran down the end of the pub together. Kids are always like that. I wonder what age you lose it. Natural friendship at first sight. And them not even drunk. Seeing who could jump the furthest on the rubber mat in front of the dartboard.

Your man's mammy looked down at them and then glanced at me. My son. My daughter. Ah, yeah. Join the club. I could see Kaya and her friend drawing on a table with a piece of yellow chalk. Third pint. Go after this one. Go.

Two lads landed in. Gary Suffin and Darren Brady. You go away for eight years and bucks still look the same only bigger and grumpier.

They slouched in behind a very pregnant girl in a Liverpool jersey and black jeans with the knees gone out of them non-fashionably. The barman looked down at the two artists near the dartboard and glanced complacently at a packet of J-Cloths. The girl in the Liverpool jersey coughed and reeled off an unravelling ball of words.

—Thanks to my fella, we don't even have money for a bag of chips. Who gave him that horse at Kilbeggan day before yesterday? Didn't matter except nothing would do him only to stick the last fiver on it.

Darren flushed and looked at a cobweb hanging near the rusty fire extinguisher behind the bar.

—Jack's Army. Fucking Jack's Army. Nearly every bob we had gone on a ticket and the trip up to Dublin.

—We're all part of Jackie's Army, Bernie.

—We are in our fuck, Darren. If he hadn't chanced the

fiver, I wouldn't have minded. Only the clothes is all stuck in the laundry now till Thursday. The smell off these jeans. I had to take this jersey off a line in the Park. And there'd be a quare niff off me only for I have these yokes.

Bernie eased up the football shirt so everyone could see the egg-shape of her pale white stomach. She reached under the belt of her jeans and pulled up a fistful of football shorts. Thwack. She snapped it against her stomach and laughed.

—We're all part of Jackie's Army.

Her absent-minded chewing of the nails on the left hand showed that her teeth should have been crowned some time. I wondered how often I should look at Kaya to see if there was anything up with her gnashers. Would I know?

—Who the fuck are you, lad?

They looked over at me. The five of them. Bernie was someone who would spend her life asking questions other people had thought about asking and then couldn't be bothered to.

—Well, I'm Bernie Sheridan, I'm fifteen.

—It's nice to meet you.

—Snazzy haircut.

—Serious jersey.

The men looked at the clock and headed for the door after a last check on the *Racing Post*. I shifted around in my stool and edged it towards the three women. It made no noise on the thick red carpet.

—I'm visiting relations. I've been in England a few years. The last time I was here, this pub wasn't.

One of the babies clutched a line of objects that hung over his head in the pram. His mother offered me a fag. I said I didn't smoke.

If you could bottle the moment when you move in from outside a group in a pub to become a part of it you'd sell a few crates to everyone. The ingredients would make sense of something none of us want to talk about.

—Where in the town are you from?

—I used be from the Park.

Kaya and her buddy came back up the pub. I flung on my jacket because I was getting too comfortable.

—You're Paul Kelly, aren't you?

The oldest of the three girls making a serious effort at being casual.

—Yeah, you have me twigged.

—Just, we're sorry about Johnny, he had a lot of friends.

—We were all mad about him.

—Stop it, Ann. You hardly remember us?

—I hardly remember anyone.

—I'm Belinda Greer, this slagbag is Ann Maloney and you know superwoman here is Bernie Sheridan.

I hadn't really forgotten them. They were fragments overheard in take-aways and amusement arcades. Bernie Sheridan's oul fella fought in Vietnam and had a steel plate in his head. The kids were taken away from him after he put the wife into Intensive Care. For the second time. Belinda Greer did a cartwheel across the Fair Green the morning I waited for the train to bring me to Dublin eight years ago. I remembered that. She waved and then a lorry came around by the corner of the Protestant church and blotted her out of sight.

Bernie ran her hand nervously across the number-nine Rush jersey before she went. She said himself would be wondering where she'd got to.

—She's some scout, said Belinda.

Ann winked at Kaya and made a face behind Belinda's back.

—You're a cunt, Ann.

—Your fucking language, young Greer.

—I better be heading, girls.

—'Bye now, said the barman without looking up as myself and Kaya hit out the door.

I turned right at the Main Street traffic lights and walked up the hill. Kaya's feet stumbled twice on cracks in the footpath. I wondered if someone had cinched the compo already. Eleven of the Rob All Reillys got a spin of the wheel over a crater on a path in the Diamond.

O'Connell Crescent in to my right. A few hundred houses and none of them with a front gate or wall. The open-plan estate. The genius who thought of that never had anyone doing a handbrake turn on his front step. A few kids played three-and-in in the middle of the road. One of them picked up the ball and looked at me as I skirted the outside of their estate and turned into Gallows Road.

No change in Gallows Road. Still a long row of houses with overgrown gardens. 'Eighty-one, 'eighty-two and 'eighty-four regs on the cars outside. Rusty vans. Terry Hannon still ran a shop without a licence. A price list in marker on a wooden board outside the front window.

A skinny black greyhound crept by us like a rat on stilts. Kaya gripped my hand. A few of the houses were boarded up. One of them had a name and number painted in white on the unvarnished wood at the front. And a skull and crossbones under the number

—Stay out. Number 38. Tony Fee, Richard Ward and Barney Devine.

An old Ford Cortina lay on its side in the front garden. The wheels were gone and someone was making a start at stripping it for scrap. Blue splotches of paint still shone surprisingly on the body. We turned down Bakers Lane. A young lad not much bigger than Kaya hammered away at a battered car bonnet on the ground.

—How are ye.

—How's it going, son.

Two fridges with the backs of them ripped out and the innards strewn around the place stood abandoned at the edge of the Lane. The Park was at the end of the Lane. This was it. People would try. But the Park would always be itself. Still no playground. Just the site of the old dump stretching out like the sea from the bottom of the Park. Uneven, overgrown and dotted with what one day were expensive new cars and the next crackling orange bonfires.

The caravans still had the wires reaching through the front windows of the relations' houses to tap into the electricity supply. Connections. The Park was all about connections.

—This is where your dad comes from, Kaya.

—Where does Granny Kelly live?

—Down the other end. Number 4. We're at Number 146.

Bernie Sheridan stood on the front step of a small white caravan and poured a saucepan of water on to the ground.

—Hello, stranger. Hello, Kaya.

—Hello, again.

—Here, catch.

Bernie dummied to throw the saucepan at me but it slid slowly from her grasp and bounced on to the footpath. I felt a lightness in my head as I bent down to pick it up. I needed three days' sleep. Bernie was taking the saucepan from me when the roar came from inside the caravan.

—Bernie, in the holy name of fuck, who are you gabbing to out there?

Clinger Clyne appeared at the door in a blue shell-suit. The same people appearing in the same places. Like eight years had been nothing and I was just walking back into my forgotten life. My old self would be waiting for me down in the house. Hanging in the wardrobe. A damp smell off it but still ready to wear.

—Well, what do you want?

—Clinger, head, how're they hangin'.

—Hang on. Jesus. Paul Kelly. You're gone as fucking stout. I'd remember you anywhere. Bernie, would you go in and keep an eye on the pan. I never trust them sausages.

—Right. Sound. See you. See you, Kaya.

Clinger jumped down on to the path.

—It's great to see you. I'm awful sorry about Johnny. This your young one?

The second sentence jammed between the first and the third like some sort of filler. Aeroboard. Sponge. We knocked off a few more sentences before I realized what I was supposed to ask him.

—Have I the wrong end of the stick or are you going to be a father yourself?

—Oh, yeah. Officially. Soon. She's a great girl. She is. We get on great. I never met a girl like her.

—You're a lucky man.

—I heard you done well for yourself. I was sorry to hear about your wife. You must have been wild cut up about it.

—It was tough for a while all right.

—You know, and people might say I'm daft, but there's been rakes more people dying of it since Chernobyl. It just shows you, doesn't it?

I wanted to say something because I knew it was my turn but I just felt my lips moving noiselessly as my head emptied. Clinger flicked eight years out of the way and pretended I'd spoken.

—We've started Colmcille United up again. Are you playing at all these days? We could do with you at centre-back.

—I wouldn't kick shite off a rope this weather. I didn't kick a ball these last four years. You'd have to play me left-back. Left back in the dressing-room.

*

Eight years since I'd seen Mam. Words. What use are they to you when you need them? At funerals and things. The right words don't exist. You know there should be right words. But when you try to say them you don't even come near. Same with actions. Never completely correct. But you don't have anything only words and actions. So you have to be going on with them. I knocked and listened. The door opened.

—How's it going, Mam.

I reached down to hug her and felt the bones of her fingers pressing into the flesh of my back. She was crying. Silently. I pulled the front door after me.

—Come on, Mam, things'll be all right.

Words. Missus Greer was in the hall.

—Ah, now, Nuala, there's no need to be crying. Sure isn't it good to see Paul home looking so well after all this time.

Oul fuck.

—And who's this big girl here? Are you going to say hello to your granny?

I take it back, Missus Greer. Kaya moved her head from side to side and brought her bottom lip up almost to her nose in one of her concentration gestures. Mam dabbed at her eyes with a white tissue from the plastic packet in her pocket before she hoisted Kaya into the air. The bones in her back clicked. Kaya gave a small scream. It must have been the sentimentalizing effect of the drink and the tiredness that made it sound the same as Lydia's scared giggle on the rollercoaster in Chessington World of Adventure.

I sat down in a chair and picked up the *Star* when the noise of the gate squeaking after Missus Greer died away. Mam's steady murmur and Kaya's rapid-fire gurgle of talk floated through from the kitchen. Then they laughed together. I threw down the paper and went out to them.

Herself and Kaya sifted through battered jigsaw boxes,

fuzzy felt kits and those yokes where you rubbed the back of a spoon against groovy paper and transferred a tiny figure on to an empty landscape. They looked through a heap of games I thought had disappeared once Johnny got old enough to leave them in the cupboard.

They didn't look at me much. I had my mind made up I didn't want to be fussed over. But I would have liked a choice. Mam came into the sitting-room when she'd put Kaya into what had been my sisters' bedroom.

—Do you want a look around the house? I have it changed a bit since you went away.

That cooker wasn't there when I went. Johnny got it. And he got her that tumble-drier a couple of Christmases ago. Liz and Tracey gave a few pounds but it was Johnny's money mostly. He put in that new range as well. The wallpaper was new. It was only a couple of years old. The kitchen was painted too.

The dodging around the house only used up a few minutes. I sat in the chair in front of the fire. Mam took the poker from the stand and dealt the briquettes a few pointless blows. Silence. I looked all around the sitting-room and then back into the fireplace.

—Who are the kids in the photos?

—They're Tracey's young ones and the ones in the photos the other side are Liz's. They have three each. I have no photograph of my other grandchild though.

I clamped the tongs around a briquette in the centre of the fire. I lifted it a few inches and dropped it back into exactly the same position.

—You've still got all the oul football trophies out as well.

—Do you remember winning that big one?

—Do I what? I still have the football bag.

The soaring sound of a firework being launched filled the next silence. We waited for the bang. Seconds. A few more unbearable waiting seconds. No finishing explosion.

—They're dangerous anyways. It's no harm. Do you want tea and a sandwich or something? Take off that shirt and put it in the wash.

She bent down to put more briquettes on the fire.

—Do you remember the way Daddy used take the orange wire off the bales with his teeth, Mam?

—I do. I remember him doing it one night when he was stocious and nearly cutting the bottom lip off himself. He had to go down to Casualty to get his mouth stitched.

—I disremember that.

Mam said she was proud of me and asked me about Lydia. I just looked into the teacup. Mam always left the teabag in. So had Lydia. It had annoyed me once. Now it was a sacred memory. I told Mam I didn't want to talk about Lydia.

—It's hard to know, Paul.

—It is. It's hard to know.

—It's only that you never sent me a wedding photo or nothing. Your sisters are still living in the Park and Johnny was always around the place. You'd think you hated home.

—Sure you can't spend your whole life living in one place.

—It never done me any harm.

—I don't suppose it did. Mam, what happened to Johnny exactly?

—He got attacked coming home from the Dandy Diner. Someone battered him with slash-hooks and stuff. He was dead when they got him to the hospital.

—Who killed him?

—No one knows. He didn't have an enemy in the world. Probably some young fellas that were high on drugs, that Ecstasy or something, they just attacked him.

—Old Bill will get them.

—Who?

—The cops. The cops'll get them.

—They say they're following a definite line of inquiry. But you'd have to be one of the poshies before that crowd would care who killed you. What odds will it make? The last thing I said to him was to mind himself. Mind yourself, son, I said to him and he just laughed the way he always laughed.

—Mam, you'll only upset yourself going on like that. Whoever did it will get sorted out one way or the other.

—Upset meself. I have enough people to do it for me. Do you want another cup of tea and something to go with it or are you going to call to Tracey and Liz for a short while? I'm going to go to bed and take something to put me to sleep.

I heard Mam out in the kitchen as I pulled the door behind me. Straightening cups on a wooden mug-tree. I was on my own in the Park. Without Johnny. It didn't feel right. Liz's house was 76. Tracey was at 70.

It was pure silent from 40 to 60. All boards and bricks over the windows and doors and a couple of signs on gates.

WARNING GUARD DOGS.

A small man in a suit walked up and down in front of Number 39 with a jet-black Alsatian on a chain in front of him. He stepped out in front of me. The dog had a growl at me and showed his teeth.

—Captain, be quiet. Don't mind him, he won't bite you. Well, there's not much way of knowing what he'd do but I don't think he'll do much when I'm here. Welcome home, Paul.

The nearest streetlamps were smashed so I couldn't see him properly although I wasn't sure if I'd know who he was anyway. He threw his hand out in the dark to me.

—Don't you remember me, man? Noelie Reilly, your brother's mate, from the Diamond.

—Noelie, how are things.

—Johnny talked a lot about you. It's good to see you. Jesus, it's desperate what happened. Ah, meself and himself were like that.

His hands swished together in the vague dark. He adjusted

44

them slightly so the fingers locked perfectly together. Knuckle joints cracked.

—I better keep going, Paul. Great to see you all the same. I'll call down to the house tomorrow. We can go for a couple of pints then.

—The removal is tomorrow.

—Oh, yeah. Yeah. See you in the church then.

Noelie. Yeah. Beetlejuice they called him. Brendan. James. Bumper. Johnny. Herbie. Marty. Bubbles. Beetlejuice. The Rob All Reillys.

The Diamond. Thirty-five houses knocked up in a fierce hurry a mile outside the town for the people who came out of the workhouse in the Twenties.

Once upon a time the men there sent their wives into the town to tempt farmers with what used be called in porno novels the delicate lotus flower of sex but was hardly that. No one from the country ever went near the Diamond any more. A good hammering and the loss of a day's money lives on in the folk memory.

The Diamond had been called Padraig Pearse Terrace but the residents took down the sign one day and replaced it with one that read Riverview Crescent. No one knew why. Or why almost everyone there was Reilly. The Rob Alls. They usually kept to themselves.

There was no answer at Number 76 and music playing in Number 70. Liz's husband Francie Boyle answered the door. He had a joint in his hand. The telly and the radio in the living-room were both on. Tracey and Liz lay on the couch with their arms round each other. Tracey's husband, Kevin McGoey, poured whiskey into mugs with faded orange-and-blue patterns on their sides.

—A little bit for you, a big bit for me. Another eentsy weentsy bit for you and il mucho biggo bitty witty for me.

—0800, look what blew in.

—0800, how goes it, dude.

o8oo because Kevin was in the army and let everyone know this by always using the twenty-four-hour clock.

—Look, Liz, the little brother is here. How the fuck are you, lad.

—Stick a joint in his gob.

—Turn off that bastarding box, someone.

Liz looked a lot older. Tracey didn't. But Liz had looked younger when they got married. Maybe because she was. The two weddings within three months of each other the year before I went to England. Francie had six stone put on. o8oo looked like he'd win back the Six Counties single-handed. In the morning.

—And a big, big drink for little bruv. And an itsy bitsy weeny teeny yellow polka-dot spliffy for me.

Ha-chaaa. Boom. Beaut. Heart slowing down a gear. Baa-daa. Baa-deeee. Calm. For the moment. Sisters. That's hard to know too. Not the same as being brothers. Unless you're a sister, I guess. Tracey giggled a lot. Liz coughed and spluttered and almost shoved the spliff light-first into the palm of my hand. Francie put his hand behind her head and held a tumbler of water to her mouth. Gently.

They didn't say much. I could see what was at the back of their eyes. Me and Johnny playing football in front of the house when we were five. Me and Johnny fishing. Johnny and me playing football for United. Johnny and me each knowing that the other would always be there to keep the eye out.

I was always going to be there to watch his back. But I hadn't been. They were thinking that and it punctured their speech balloons before they even hit the air.

The telly got turned back on. The Superstars of Wrestling cavorted around silently. o8oo was up beside it with his ears glued to the lowered volume. Tracey was asking me questions about England when Liz let a yelp out of herself and sat up dead straight.

46

—Johnny is dead. He's dead so he is and we'll never see him again.

0800's voice was reedy as if he was on the verge of breaking into tears.

—Who do you think killed him?

—I don't know. It's, like, you hear stories, you know, a few different things.

—But you know this town for rumours.

—Do ye have any clue?

Every footstep out in the Park seemed heading for that front door. Johnny should come in, throw his coat over the couch, tease Tracey about her hair and we'd slap our hands together in the air. He was out there but he couldn't come in.

—Would ye ever talk about something else, would ye? Ye're so interested in that sort of shite.

Liz's voice silenced the three of us. Tracey looked over at me. Her and Liz huddled together at the edge of the couch. Our distance from them embarrassed us, I think.

—Paul, how come you didn't bring your kid down here, how? How come you left her at home, how? You'd never think we'd be interested. You never even told us her name.

Tracey said they knew it was Kaya.

—I never heard him say it.

I was between sleep and half awake. 0800 was saying he thought it was people from outside the town. Out-of-town sham job was the odds.

—I definitely heard in the barracks it was an outside gang. If meself and Francie knew who it was . . .

Some fear but more anger buzzed off Tracey's voice.

—You'd do what? You'd do nothing. I'll tell you something for nothing, whoever was able to kill my brother would handle you.

—I can look after meself.

—No, you can't. You know you can't. If Johnny Kelly can't then nobody can.

—Come over tomorrow and see Kaya, I said, though I knew it wasn't relevant to the conversation.

Tracey put her arm around me and pulled my head into the warmth of her shoulder. I could feel my eyes closing as I smelt wool and the remnants of a perfume that smelt like flowers freshly pressed between scrapbook pages. Francie's voice was floating somewhere above me. Curious.

—I saw him a bit before it happened, you know. He was in a snug in the Dandy Diner just before closing time. Talking to someone but I couldn't see who it was. I could only see his back. He left the place a few minutes later. And that was Johnny.

And that was Johnny. In the morning I woke and found I had staggered back across the Park to sleep the night in my old room. My old room. And Johnny's. I wanted to tell him I loved him and this wouldn't be the end of things. But I knew he'd left me. Him and all.

Three

They're Absolutely Ooky

Mam had left an alarm clock beside the bed. I don't know why. I tried to stop the ringing. And the jangling. It jumped up and down on the bedside table before I found the off button.

Bells and alarms. One March 18th morning Lydia shot out a skinny arm, picked up a ringing clock and fucked it against the wall in one athletic movement. It smashed to smithereens. I laughed until my left side started paining me. Vinnie bought us a replacement. An alarm clock in the shape of a little Samurai warrior who shouted at you every morning in Japanese.

Kaya went through a stage when I'd have to set your man to go off a dozen times a day. She'd move up very near to it and then give a wet scream of kiddy laughter as he started his spiel. His glockenspiel.

—Hitachi Fuji Yokohama Sushi Karaoke Nissan Emperor Hirohito Kurosawa You Lazy Bastard.

Or something like that.

Mam was delicately removing the contents of a Quinnsworth Breakfast Pack when I hit the kitchen. Sausages, rashers and black puddings.

—There's cereal there if you want it. I got one of them variety packs because I didn't know what kind Kaya likes.

She flipped an egg over. The bacon spat. She quickly shook her hand.

—How come you don't have your car home with you?

—Bagged. Bagged and banned. Another six months to go.

Mam cracked another egg in the pan and shook her head the way she used to when one of us got the bum's rush out of school.

—That's bad now, Paul. It's a gammy chant.

—It's cuck melodeon, Mam.

—Cutmaloda.

Kaya put her hand up to her mouth the way she did when she wasn't sure if it was a good word or a bad word. The odd time.

—It's all right, Kaya. It's Irish. Gaelic. Show your granny your good Irish.

—*Kaya O Kyalee is amin dom.*

—Good girl. Does she learn it in school over there?

—Does she fuck. I taught her that. She can count up to ten in Bengali though.

Kaya finally settled on Coco Pops. Again. I still think there's something not quite right about them. And she had to sing that fucking song.

—I'd rather have a bowl of Coco Pops. Yes, I'd rather have a bowl of Coco Pops. We'd rather have a bowl of Co-o-co Pops.

I picked up another packet and tapped her on the side of the nose with it.

—Would you not prefer these, Kaya? You know. Snap, crackle and pop, snap, crackle and pop, snap, crackle and pop, snap, crackle and pop.

Mam looked over at me and tapped her ring finger against her forehead. She still wore her wedding ring. The oul fella probably melted his down and sold it to Brendan Stokes for scrap before he headed for the hills.

—You're daft. Do you know that? Show some respect for your dead brother.

—Ah, Mam, come on. All these oul ad tunes are great. You'll give us a few bars.

I walked into the kitchen, caught her around the waist and took the spatula in my left hand.

—Come on down and sing into the mike. You're on stage with the Cotton Mill Boys in the Temperance Hall. Sing. Or I'll tickle you. This used to be the National Anthem around here, Kaya. You do the Shake 'n' Vac and put the freshness back/Do the Shake 'n' Vac and put the freshness back/When your carpet smells fresh your room does tooo-oo-oo/Every time you shake it remember what to do.

Mam laughed. Kaya's spoon was arrested halfway between bowl and mouth. Off-white milk tinged with brown dripped on to the table.

—Cutmaloda.

—No, no, Kaya, wikkid.

—Wikkid. Kickin'.

Mam took the spatula out of my paw and set her face back in its frown.

—You're still drunk. Remember you're home for a funeral. Ye'll all end up dead the way ye drink. Sit down at the table and I'll give you your breakfast.

I swiped a cloth and wiped up the spillage from Kaya's spoon. Kaya slurped the milk from the bottom of the bowl. I took a tissue and wiped the milk drops and the little Coco Pops flakes from her mouth.

—Eat that fry now, Paul, or you'll get an ulcer from drinking and not eating. I don't know why ye don't look after yere health when ye have a choice in the matter.

I heard her gulp when she closed the back door behind her. Her arms were full of little plastic bags of sticks when she came back in.

—You could have let me do that, Mam.

—You wouldn't know where anything is.

She switched on the toaster and dipped a Silk Cut into the bowels of the machine until it lit. Her thumb switched the toaster off again. A second later her ring finger flicked on the radio. Gaybo's wheedling tones zoomed out across Dublin, nipped through Kilmainham, got stuck in a traffic jam in Maynooth, bombed out as far as Kinnegad, had a bite to eat in Harry's and took the Mullingar bypass to avoid the traffic lights before taking their perennial place in the Kelly family kitchen.

Absence hadn't made my heart grow any fonder of the oul bastard. I went out to the sitting-room because I saw Mam wanted to start talking about Johnny again. Kaya asked me to give her five.

—To the left, to the right, down below, too slow.

I pretended to be surprised when she pulled her hand away. Mam walked into the room with three mugs of coffee on a tray.

—Does she like coffee?

There was no stopping her talking about Johnny. It was all that stopped her crying about him. She asked me if I knew who Gazza was. I said I did. Johnny was obsessed with him, she said. Wore the same clothes. Had his hair cut the same way. Wore the same football gear as him. Even changed his boots when Gazza signed a new sponsorship deal. Even played like him, Clinger told her. Ponced around midfield and tried to beat four players on a run every few minutes. Never hit the ball straight when he could curl it.

—Is there anything wrong with Gazza, Paul?

—Nothing notable. Nothing that can't be cured.

—It's only I overheard someone in Quinnsworth the other day saying that if Johnny hadn't been at that Gazza crack he might still be alive.

—That was only them being nasty. There's no reason anyone would want to kill Gazza. That was only spite talking. You'll always have that.

—He was mad on the chap, Paul. A couple of Sundays he was here and Glasgow Rangers were playing. He made me sit down and watch it and look at everything Gazza did.

Liz and Tracey and their six sprogs landed in at noon. It wasn't till they arrived I realized how quiet the house had been. Mam would live in that silence from now on.

Tracey winked at me and fussed over Kaya. Liz lit the next cigarette off the butt of the last one. And I was Uncle Paul to six kids. Suddenly. Brian, Claudine and Stella McGoey and Jennifer, Robbie and Johnny Boyle.

Liz's two eldest stayed beside their mother. Baby Johnny kept a cracking monologue going in his pram.

—Gagagaga, gaga, gagaaa, ga ga ga ga ga ga ga gag ga.

I don't know why but I did the penny-lifted-from-behind-the-ear trick on Stella.

—D'you know what, Liz, Johnny sounds just like his dad.

The nieces and nephews decided Kaya wanted to go for a walk. The McGoeys pulled out of her like she was a Scalextric that wouldn't last till Stephen's Morning. The Boyles walked along behind them. Liz talked out in the kitchen. I could hear Mam listening. It was something to do with the stillness around the space that held Liz's voice as though it was a glass taw stuck in the neck of a bottle.

—You shouldn't let her be waiting on you hand and foot. It's not good for her, she's very tired these days, Tracey said to me.

Tracey's voice was glass too. Hard. Clear. Concern scratched the surface and spoiled the perfect appearance.

—She's all right. I didn't ask her to do anything. You know what she's like, she likes doing things.

—She doesn't, you know. She only does them because she thinks she has to.

Tracey joined the other two women in the kitchen and soon I heard the three of them talking. Mainly Liz's voice with the pitch changing every few sentences. Tracey chiding. Mam chipping in monosyllables but mainly listening. Listening and concentrating.

The Angelus was bong-bonging good-o when I saw Uncle Jimmy approaching the front door. He blew into the palm of his hand and sniffed the breath with interest. The collar was being straightened when I opened the door.

—Jesus Christ, the young lad himself. Home is the sailor, home from the sea. Stand up there till I get a look at you.

—I am standing up. Come in, y'oul bollocks, before you frighten the neighbours.

Jimmy waited for me to sit down on the chair before he perched on the edge of the couch. He rubbed his hands together like he was trying to eliminate them by erosion. When he was the Rovers goalie he used rub chewing gum on those hands before a game because he reckoned this would make the ball stick to them.

—Paul, you wouldn't, you know, be able to let me have a whatyoumaycall, oul *gruaig* of the dog job like. Jesus, would you look at these hands.

I didn't know whether the shake was real or whether he was acting up.

—There's an oul bottle of Jameson in the small press behind you.

The helpful voice on him. The bottle was half empty. Or half full. The optimist and the pessimist. Wonder if that means anything. It sat on top of a big jigsaw box with a picture of a castle on it. Kenilworth Castle I think it was. Jimmy brought it back from England.

He travelled all over England and Ireland. At the three-card trick. Himself and a gyp called Johnny Cash. Johnny Cash got killed in a big tinker fight in Donegal in the Sixties and Jimmy packed the trick in. He had a tattoo on his left shoulder. JAMES AND ROSE FOR EVER.

A heart with an arrow piercing it from the side, a sword going down through the middle and a snake with its tongue out wrapped around the sword. Even Mam, Jimmy's favourite sister, hadn't a notion who Rose was or had been. There seemed to be something in Jimmy's eyes when he was asked about it. But he'd done the three-card trick for too many years for you to trust his eyes.

His body kicked forward when he swallowed the first drop of whiskey. One o'clock. In six hours we'd be in Reynolds' Funeral Home and Johnny's body would be removed to the Cathedral.

—Will you come for a pint?

Jimmy's voice came out of the corner of his mouth as usual. I was putting on my jacket when Tracey looked in the door and told me to make sure Jimmy didn't stay too long in Donoghue's and didn't get too drunk before the removal. Oul fucker Jimmy asked me for a sub before we even got to Donoghue's and said he'd sort me out tomorrow. It made me think of the sign Lydia bought for behind the bar in the King William. FREE BEER TOMORROW.

Donoghue's was changed fuck-all from when I crawled around under the stools. Joe still had that big red book behind the bar with the names of everyone from the Park who was drinking on tick. Thick stubby iron bars had appeared in front of the small windows since I was here last. Inside had the murky light of a darkroom. A curly-haired woman with an English accent broke off from chatting to a couple of old-timers when we walked in.

—All right, James.

—All right, Sharon, still getting it wet?

—Don't be a git, James. Usual?

—Aye and a pint of porter for the child. Git, that's a great oul word.

People kept coming over to try and console us. All of them struggling to find the right face and the right words. I made a half-hearted move to pull on my jacket when the little hand reached three. Jimmy grabbed me by the shoulder.

—Hang on a minute. We'll just have a couple more. You know how it is.

I knew how it was. How it is. But I still leaned on a quotation sneaked out of a library book that said you couldn't be an alcoholic until you were thirty. Alcoholic was a daft word anyways. It belonged to the men in grey suits who turned up at Second Mass to tell you they'd lost their businesses because of the drink but Jesus had helped them and now they were happy.

Some mornings you expect Skylab to fall on your head. Or a big lump of green ice flushed out of a jumbo jet jacks.

Another pint. With a whiskey chaser this time. Jimmy's face glowed. My heart jumped as it decided whether to settle or not.

Jimmy ordered another round. Sharon went to write it down in the book. I flung a mangled sterling tenner on to the counter.

—Look at me, I'm not mean, digging trenches for the Queen.

One Monday I was reading the magazine of one of those Sundays Kerrie buys to read reviews of plays and films. She never gets to see them because she won't go without me. This English writer reckoned there's this tribe out in Africa or somewhere who are pissed the whole fucking time. They have no problem, your man reckons, because they think it's natural to be constantly langered.

Only they probably think it's natural to be jumping ten foot up in the air every time you hear a small noise. Except that might be handy if you were out in the jungle because you'd never get eaten by a lion. Even the cross-eyed one that was in *Daktari*. You'd be safe enough the whole time, of course, with Snagglepuss who I'd say is a vegetarian sort of a skin of a lion.

That pint must have cooled it. I was thinking about cartoons.

I'd be farting them later.

Mary Ann McDonagh joined us. Her husband was out looking for a stray greyhound. She picked a jam doughnut off the counter and cut it in two. Mary Ann nibbled half-heartedly and talked to Jimmy about when the Galway Races were the real Galway Races and people had time for each other.

People had stopped reading the *Irish Press* in pubs since I'd been away. Simon McDonagh walked in and said something despairing. Himself and Mary Ann owed the Council £3,000 in back rent. They were preparing to go back on the side of the road. The Health Board offered to put them up in hospital but Simon and Mary Ann would have to be separated from each other if that happened so they turned down the offer. Simon told her not to worry about the greyhound. He couldn't run fast enough to get anywhere too far away.

—He ain't nothin' but a hound dog.

Jimmy was gone very comical in himself the last few minutes and looked like he was going to launch into some ballad about Rathbawn's Noble Ten. I decided it was time to get him home and left half a pint at the counter so I'd feel better about myself.

Stepping into the light and the air was like stepping out of a cinema after watching *Gone with the Wind*. Twice. Woooosh. Bullshit, haaah. We straightened up and shivered and walked down Gallows Road as if we were floating above it. My feet hit every crack in the footpath. And there were enough. Jimmy fell asleep on his couch the minute I got him in the door.

I thought of Kaya on my way back from Jimmy's. Wondering how much she'd remember of this. The first memory I have is of an FA Cup final in black-and-white when I was four. There's no way she can remember anything from when she was not even two. She can't remember Lydia. She can't. No way.

Rough the way I keep thinking of Kaya. Wondering who she thinks like. Me? Lydia? There's something about character traits skipping a generation. Like the way you're more tired the second day after a batter. I think of myself as a kid. Fear and loneliness and so on as well as the good stuff. All this in store for her.

You can't but think they'll turn out the same way as yourself. Same joys. Same sadnesses. I have that worry that Kaya will some day feel how I do these mornings. She will look down and say whose are these hands and whose are these feet and what am I doing with them. I am more scared of that than of anything else. You can calm down and make yourself put these thoughts out of your own mind. You can block them out. But you can't be in someone else's head. Even if you love them. I found that out.

It's the dirtiest trick of all. Making you watch a smaller version of yourself walking down the same path. And letting you know you can do sweet fuck-all about it. Except carry them on your shoulders while they're still light enough.

'Eddie Clyne, Car Dismantlers, Gallows Road, Rathbawn.'

Gold writing on the side of a black car parked where Gallows Road turned into Bakers Lane. A Saab Turbo. Three phone numbers. Clinger's a canny brother.

Eddie was leaning against the bonnet. Talking into a mobile phone. He'd dyed the hair blond sometime over the last eight years. The phone call finished when I was ten yards away from the car. He looked nervy. Like he knew my face but wasn't definite on who I was. I recognized him before he recognized me. It was the first time that had happened. I stuck out the paw. We gave each other the crush-the-bones shake. The scrap business obviously gave you muscles like a gym-trained mountain gorilla.

—Aaaaah. Are you not talking to the people now you've your money made, you bad bastard?

—From what we heard I have a bit to go yet to catch up with you, you yuppie. Sit in for a chat. Oh, and sorry for your troubles. I mean it.

Eddie's car phone rang. He raised a hand apologetically and slapped the receiver against his ear.

—Yeah. Yeah. Who? Yeah. Fuck him. Around half an hour. Put it in the microwave sure when I get home. An hour maybe. I have to see Willie Kett at the yard. If anyone calls say I'm busy. I'm talking to Paul Kelly. Yeah. Poor oul Johnny's brother. Right. Yeah.

He pressed a button and then left the phone off the hook. The gesture had love twined around it. Like a king cobra.

—Sorry about that. The wife. You'd think I was a hundred miles away from her or something.

—Oh, yeah. Congrats. I heard you got kettled to Dalton Dunbar's little sis.

—Thanks. Yeah. Sonia. Well it makes you feel you're not doing it all for nothing. Great woman. Funky chick, you know.

He sounded happy but he frowned a lot.

—I hear you're coining it at the oul scrap this weather.

Eddie chewed a protruding edge of nail on his left little finger.

—Yeah. It's not going bad. Long oul hours. And the money is all cash into the hand so you spend a lot more than you think. I heard you're flying it beyond.

—Sort of. Same as yourself. If I stopped it'd all disappear.

—How's your mother? Will she get over it?

—She'll get by. The woman is the world champ of getting by. She could give talks on it. I met Clinger yesterday evening.

All those words did was make Eddie look sad. And tired. There was a shrug of the shoulders in his face.

—Ah, yeah. Gerry is Gerry. I'm trying to fix him up with something this ages. But you can do nothing for him. He won't work with me and he won't take anything from me.

Eddie and Clinger refused to play on opposing teams in the National School yard. Then they refused to pass the ball to each other.

—He seems happy enough.

—Suppose. We can all do little enough for our brothers really. The only thing Gerry ever took off me was a set of jerseys for that football team of his. The same boys wouldn't win a game of blow football in an oxygen tent. I'll give you a lift down home.

The commiseration was so thick in the sitting-room you could hardly see your hand in front of your face. Relations and half-relations and neighbours. Kaya sitting on Mam's knee.

—All right, Dad.

—All right, pet. She hasn't been any trouble, Mam?

—Not a bit. I'll tell you something for nothing, she's in the ha'penny place for trouble compared to you at the same age. Meself and herself are getting on like a house on fire.

The head wasn't great. Noisy cogwheels seemed to be

grinding in it. Lie down. Yeah. Lie down. You can always lie down.

I could have had a lie-down on my old bed but Liz had me beaten to it. She was fully dressed. Her hands were clasped behind her head. She looked up at the ceiling. So did I. But I couldn't see anything.

—It's shite, isn't it?

Liz pulled the syllables out slowly like someone dragging a deep lake. A black dark deep lake.

—What is?

—It all. The whole crack. It's shite.

Her face was fierce blotchy and fierce red. She sat up and shook herself. Then she balled up her fists and rubbed them against her eyes. Viciously. She blinked when she took them away and shook her head.

—No, it's still the same shite.

She flopped on to her back when I sat down beside her. The bed creaked. In the hall Robbie roared because Jennifer had hit him a clip he'd been putting out for. I told Liz Johnny wouldn't have wanted her to be like this about his death. It crossed my mind it wouldn't have crossed Johnny's mind he was going to die. Liz giggled. It was a horrible laugh. Like one forced out of her by some gang who were holding her hostage. To show she was in good health and being well treated.

—If it was only the funeral I wouldn't feel that bad. But I don't know if I feel sad about him getting killed. Because I feel sad all the time.

Her fingers plaited and unplaited the same strands of hair as she talked.

—Do you ever get the bubble, Paul? When it's building up inside you all day and you're waiting for it to pop but it doesn't and it just keeps getting bigger.

—'Course I do. Everyone gets depressed. You're not the only one, Liz.

—D'you ever see blood coming out of the walls?

—What? No. Don't be daft.

—Well, I have. A lock of times. And then Mam has to look after the kids. I seen blood coming out of the walls of every room in the house. Once it was just one room, the living-room, and if I went and sat in another room it would be OK. But now when it starts it's every room. In anyone's house. I'm a fucking loonybin is what I am.

I couldn't think of a shtime to say to her. I knew the edges of what she was on about. But that was all.

—I hear voices too. I go into the kitchen because I'm purely convinced I hear people I know talking there. And not a sinner in it.

She rolled over to the other side of the bed and pulled her legs up into her chest. Then she kneaded the bedspread the way Kaya used do with an old blue-and-white blanket Kerrie eventually persuaded her to get rid of.

—D'you know, I say a prayer every night to Dr Roche or Mr Roche or whoever Roche is. Only for Roche Fives I'd be floating down the canal this long time.

—You sound like a fucking ad for them. Nine out of ten housewives prefer Roche Fives. It's the honeycombed middle that weighs so little.

—Fuck off, will you, Paul. D'you know what the poshies call this estate, do you? Pill Hill. Only for Roche Fives the street outside would be full with people running around screaming their heads off. Are you wide to that, are you?

—Sorry, I didn't mean to make a joke of it.

Liz pulled a pillow over her head. It muffled her voice.

—Why not? A joke is what it is.

I stood there for a few seconds and then I walked out of the room. Jennifer sat outside in the hall with Kaya on her lap. She looked at me. I tried not to look at her. Liz shouted from the bedroom.

—Jen, would you ever go down to Hannon's and buy me

a pair of tights. Opaque tights. Remember that like a good girl.

Jennifer let Kaya off her lap. I wanted to get out of the house. I felt like a trap was being set for me. I wanted to go somewhere and Terry Hannon's shop would do. I'd think of something else to do when I came back and then it would be time for the removal and then it would nearly be night.

This house wasn't mine. My mother owned the keys. She owned the sadness too. It made me feel eighteen again. The day was gone like a repeat showing of a film I'd never wanted to see in the first place.

It felt like there was something I had to do for Johnny. To make me believe he had been alive. The thought had followed me across on the boat. I couldn't stop it. Maybe it would stay in the house if I went into the fresh air.

—Liz, myself and Kaya will go. Do you want anything else?

—How can you go? What would you know about tights?

—Enough. I was married, you know.

A sewage pipe had come uncovered in Bakers Lane. It funnelled uncensored shit on to the surface of the lane. The Council wouldn't do anything about it till someone slipped and hurt themselves. And sent in the solicitor's letter. They'd fix it then. And crib later when they had to pay the compo.

Kaya was singing the same song over and over again. I hadn't heard her sing it before. She must have picked it up from her cousins. The oral tradition. I wonder is Friggin' in the Riggin' still to be had.

> Glory Glory Alleluia
> The teacher hit me with a ruler
> The ruler turned red
> And the teacher dropped dead
> Now there ain't no school no more.
> Glory Glory what a hell of a way to die

Glory Glory what a hell of a way to die
Glory Glory what a hell of a way to die
And there ain't no school no more.

A gang of young lads wheeled Quinnsworth trolleys and tractor tyres down Gallows Road. They flew past us. The rattle of the trolleys over the bumps in the road made me grit my teeth. I nipped the tip of my tongue. Two of them lingered behind to try and put the bite on us. They looked about ten. Or eight. Hard to tell at that age. Especially when you're trying to avoid eye contact.

—Mister, mister, would you have fifty pence for us? Go on, mister, you have some change.

The ten- or eight-year-olds kept walking in front of us, skipping ahead and dodging from side to side as if one of my ears might be more sympathetic than the other. All the while jabbering in the staccato style of a short-tempered dealer trying to offload a particularly crap beast at Rathbawn mart.

—Mister, mister, give us some money, please.

—Mister, mister, you have the bobs. Good man.

—Mister, we'll sing a song for you.

Glory Glory Man. United
Glory Glory Man. United
Glory Glory Man. United
And the Reds go marching on on on.

The last three words came out as
—Uh uh uh.
—Sorry, lads, I'm a Liverpool fan.

Glory Glory Liverpoo-oo-l
Glory Glory Liverpoo-oo-l
Glory Glory Liverpoo-oo-l
And the Reds go marching on on on.

Uh. Uh. Uh. I gave the bigger of the two lads a quid coin. He snapped a snot-streaked hand shut on it and sprinted down towards Hannon's.

—What about me? He won't give me any of that.

The smaller lad sounded hopeful but I think he realized. He tore after his buddy. The baggy shorts reached halfway down his legs to a pair of knees more plastered than George Best on a bad night.

—They're daft, said Kaya before restarting her own singing with a new number.

They're spooky, they're kooky
They're absolutely ooky
Dookey dookey dookey
The Addams Family
Da-da de-de de-de
Da-da de-de de-de
Da-da de-de da-da de-de da-da de-de de-de de-de.

She sang it a couple of times and tried to click her fingers when they were supposed to be clicked. But she couldn't.

—Dad, can you click your fingers?

—Yes. I can.

—Go on then. Click them.

I suddenly felt nervous and cracked the upper joints of my fingers to make them more. More. What's my word? More clicky. Kaya stood still. So did I. In front of Number 67 Gallows Road.

I held my hand at eye-level for Kaya. And wondered when was the last time I clicked my fingers. I couldn't think. I had a feeling it was a trick I couldn't master in National School. And there hadn't been much call for finger-clicking since. In fact I wasn't sure if I'd ever produced the proper snapping sound from my fingers. I tried a couple of times. It was no cinch. My hands were all slippy with sweat. I looked at Kaya.

She looked back. Unmoved. The sound of skin rubbing against skin didn't convince her. I tried again. No dice. Again. *Kerrrach. Yesssss.* Fucking A. Great one. Kaya laughed and punched me on the knee.

—Do it again, Dad.

—Ah, no, come on. We better get to the shop.

The pain was still throbbing in my thumb when we walked into Hannon's. Terry himself slouched over the counter. The brown boxes with the tins of beans, packets of crisps and twenty fags were even further behind the counter. The most resourceful kid couldn't shoplift from him now. You'd have to break into the shop.

He sorry-for-your-troubled me quickly before dealing with the two scuts who'd blodged the quid. Terry handed them out a couple of home-made fireworks from a box under the counter lined with brown paper. They scooted after he threw in a box of matches for free. I looked at Terry. Terry shrugged his shoulders.

—Fuck them. They'll be robbing this place every night in a couple of years.

Four

Something Like Vinegar

Beetlejuice was in the sitting-room with a glass in his hand and a Slim Panatella in his gob when I got back. He catapulted out of the chair, put the glass down and shook hands with me. The paw slapped out so eagerly I half expected a joy-buzzer on it.

—We meet again, hah. The women is getting ready. Your mother is a great oul fighter, do you know that? Jesus, it's unbelievable about Johnny. Uuuuunbelievable.

Then he hugged me. A great steam of stale drink off his breath. I knew it was off his breath because I was holding mine. He was sniffing. Really. Actual genuine fucking bona fide guaranteed Irish tears.

—Fuck's sake. What are we going to do without him? He was the real thing, Paul. He was the real thing.

I moved a couple of steps back and

unwound his arm from my shoulder. It wasn't hard because the arm was soft. Soft and limp and dragging like a weed catching you in Derrynagun Woods where Uncle Jimmy used bring myself and Johnny to shoot foxes. He sold the pelts.

Kids were playing rattle-tin on the wasteground. I looked out the window at them. Beetlejuice's grief made me embarrassed for him. No. That's another lie. It made me embarrassed for me. Like I still didn't feel sorry enough about Johnny. Beetlejuice was trying to smile when I looked back. He filled a shot glass with clear liquid from a Sanor Raspberry Cordial bottle.

—Poitin. You'll have a drop. Just a small drop before the removal. It's good stuff. If it wasn't, I'd be blind this long time.

Beetlejuice handed me the glass. It was all purely daft. I'd never spoken two words to this cunt in my natural. He threw his drink back in one. A funny style of drinking. The glass got brought to the right corner of his mouth and the drink was angled down that side. He twigged me looking at that. The Rob Alls were always dead wide.

—The teeth are all rotten down the other side. Killing me. I'll have to see the dentist next week. I'd be there already but they're all butchers in this town. Fucking savages. They shouldn't be let out.

What time was it? Half six. I peeked at the clock and wished I could think of something to say to him. A couple of questions about how come he was so friendly with Johnny were roller-blading across the brain-box but they wouldn't translate into words.

—It's just, Paul, if you or your mother or any of the family need help, just ask me, right? Anything at all I can do to help. An oul lift to the Cathedral or anything.

I was going to tell him we were OK but thanks all the same only what the fuck is it to you and where in the name of the Third Secret of Fatima did you buy those white slip-ons and I hope you still have the name of the fuckdog that sold them to you. But before I could, he jumped out of his chair like the angry man in the back row of a chat-show audience.

You would have sworn he'd gone through the three doors to the back yard without touching them if he hadn't left the second one open.

Someone knocked at the front door. I could see the squad parked outside. People in the Park stopped talking in their front gardens and looked into ours. Mam's yell.

—Liz, will you get that?

Liz's voice wobbled a wee bit. As if she was straining to hit a note that was out of her range.

—I'm getting Kaya dressed. Could you not get it, Mam?

I got it. Two cops. One a detective. The other a bluebottle called Cosgrave who came from Mayo and trained under-age Gaelic teams.

—Do you mind if we come in? It's only for a minute.

—Fire ahead. It's the guards, Mam. We're trying to get ready for the removal, boys. D'ye want to come into the kitchen?

Beetlejuice's glasses of poitín still sat in the sitting-room. The bottle stood to attention in front of the fireplace. They'd hardly do us for it this day. They would and all. For the crack.

Cosgrave sat across the kitchen table from me. The other boyo was definitely a detective. He had to be. They all wore those smart-casual jackets no matter where the fuck they were. And crap plain ties along with them.

The detective walked around the kitchen and studied the pictures on the walls. There's some film or telly tec does that. Cops are pure obsessed with the box and the movies. They seem to use them as training videos. Why? Imagine me behind the bar of the King William using the old Tom

Cruise in *Cocktail* technique. Hey-ooop. Flipping those bottles of Stone's Ginger Wine and Gold Label head over heels for the old codgers who come in and tell you they were stationed in Northern Ireland in the Second World War, like you give a shit.

The dynamic duo asked me a few daft questions and said they'd be off and to tell Mam they'd called. They didn't call her Mam, naturally enough.

—Any word on who killed my brother?

—We were following a definite line of inquiry but we're not making much progress at this moment in time.

Cosgrave sounded like he was listing the serial numbers of stolen television sets on *Garda Patrol*.

—There's not a lot we can do. There's very little we can be expected to do, in fact. These things seem to be part of the culture down here, don't they?

Even the way the detective closed the door had a dig in it.

Francie drove us to the funeral home. I felt I was dreaming the journey at five in the morning. I was glad I was jarred. Then, you're always glad you're when you are jarred. The hassle is the afters.

People looked into the coffin. All awkward. None of them knowing how they were supposed to act. Uncle Jimmy twisted a black hat in his hands like he was trying to wring it bone-dry. Mam started roaring and the hat rolled across the floor and came to rest at my feet as Jimmy pulled her back from the coffin. The black hat stood the right way up. As if a man was wearing it and would rise up through that cold floor. Jimmy was kept too busy wrestling with Mam to ask for his hat back.

—The last thing I said to him was to mind himself. The last thing I said to him. Oh, it was the last thing I said.

Not a mark on Johnny's face. Two blue bumps on either side of his head all right. But his face was perfect. He'd been laid out in a Tottenham Hotspur jersey. Gazza.

He did look a bit like Gazza. But the haircut probably had something to do with that.

The hair keeps growing when you're dead. Goes into overdrive when you're in the grave. So he'd look like Ruud Gullit soon enough. This whole wooden box job. Gammy chant.

0800 stood in front of the coffin and had a couple of words with everyone as they came in. He had to be doing guard duty on something. Stella McGoey was roaring, bawling, fucking demented crying. Tracey had a thin blue line running from the left corner of her mouth to her chin. You could only see it when she lost the rag. It nearly jumped out of her face now. She lifted Stella up. Stella gave a couple of feeble kicks. Tracey's words sounded like they were ground out from somewhere between her teeth and her nose.

—Get up there now, good girl, and kiss your Uncle Johnny goodbye.

The kid tried to draw back. Shrinking back, I think is what you'd call it. Putting her hands over her eyes and flinching as if she could in some way disappear back through herself. Tracey's face didn't change one muscle of expression. She didn't look to the left. She didn't look to the right. Just took Stella's hands down and lowered her so she could kiss that white, waxy, shop-window imitation-fruit face. Stella's face was whiter again when Tracey brought her away.

Kaya didn't know what was going on. She just messed with her corn-row. Tracey looked over at me and made small movements with her head. I didn't cop. Until I noticed she was contorting her face so one eye looked at Kaya, the other at the coffin and half of each at me. No. No way. Leave it out. What did Sarf Londoners say? I'm not wearing it. I wasn't wearing this. Tracey shuffled around the back of the family circle.

—I think you should bring Kaya up to look at Johnny.

—You're joking, aren't you? Ha ha. What a funny one.

—It's only right. The other kids kissed him.

—Well, that's other kids. You do what you want with yours but my daughter's got enough to put up with.

She said a few more things but I just blanked her out and watched her opening and closing her mouth without saying anything. I blanked her out like I would have a drunk shouting at me across the counter of the King William. Which made me feel guilty for the second before I remembered why I never came home. Families and your own place have you every way. All you can do is think of your other life.

I looked out a Glasgow hotel window at two in the morning after my wedding. At people in suits staggering around a carpark and wondering had they driven or walked to the reception. That day I finally reckoned I'd reached a definite destination from which I could map out the rest of my life. From which we could map out the rest of our lives. Lydia draped gauzy arms around my shoulders as I looked out that window.

—What you thinking about, love?

—Happiness and all the other stuff like that.

—I thought you were thinking about the pub and wondering if Vinnie's cleaned the lines properly.

—Nah.

—I bet y'are now.

—Be quiet, Missus Kelly. I'm thinking how I've finally made an honest woman out of you.

—I've always been an honest woman.

Did she really say that? Or have I imagined it? Embellished it. Touched it up with the old significance airbrush. So that down the road it makes sense of something. Like a line muttered early on in a whodunnit that holds the key to the entire bamboozling conundrum.

None of my family were at the wedding. They got a few postcards from Limassol to tell them it was over. A good few of our regulars landed up to Glasgow. When you've heard one Chelsea fan asking a bagpiper what's under his kilt you've heard them all.

Lydia was working in the Duke of Cambridge when I walked in there on my second day in London. Looking for a job. The pub sagged at the bottom of a block of flats in NW6. Behind it was an estate where buses wouldn't stop and where postmen wouldn't deliver any envelopes containing anything valuable.

There wasn't an iota between us first. I was in London to stay out of jail. Lydia's story had to do with a married man whose in-laws favoured a hands-on approach to preserving the family unit. Both of us were learning the pub trade. And learning to deal with the varied and challenging nature of the job the brewery goes on about in the recruitment brochure.

We dealt with it stoically. Sort of. To tell you the truth, Marcus Aurelius would have found it difficult enough to handle. I got twenty stitches in my head after a young lad hit me with a meat-cleaver because he was having trouble locating his Afro-Caribbean identity in the context of colonialist British society. Another scumbag made shit out of Lydia's arm with an iron bar because she tried to stop him making off with the till in the middle of the night. Her forearm would always crack slightly when she turned over at seven in the mornings to grab the Teasmade.

I can still feel surprised about how good I felt the day she walked into the Flock of Swans. Three weeks after I'd landed there as assistant manager. She acted surprised. Said she didn't know this was where I'd been moved to. But she couldn't keep that up for even an hour. Lydia was crap at telling lies. Always. Always.

Myself and Lydia were some operators. The perfect pair. The Batman and Robin. The Bonnie and Clyde. The Gilbert and Sullivan. I said that to Vinnie one day. He said:

—And?

—How do you mean?

—And?

—What do you mean and?

—Gilbert O'Sullivan and who?

We moved in jig time from one hand-painted sign over a varnished door to another. From long-necked swans in a blue sky to a train at a station to a fierce-looking black bull to a stable-boy tending a chestnut mare. Every sign had less chips gone off it. Every door had a newer gloss. The Horse and Groom was our first pub as a management couple. Next came the King William.

'One of the flagship pubs of the company and a major challenge for an ambitious young couple.' The brochure was telling us how far we'd come.

O'Neill, Genghis Khan of brewery area managers, called down to the King William during our first week. He couldn't believe how well we'd done. We were his protégés, he said. The way he pronounced it, it rhymed with dee-jays.

The punters threw a party for us on our final night in the Horse and Groom. O'Neill turned up *en route* to a nightclub opening in Bromley. He sang 'The Rose of Tralee' and disappeared back into a hired limousine. On his way out he deposited two bottles of Moët & Chandon behind the counter in a white plastic bag. It was the first time he'd ever given anyone a present, he told us.

We opened that champagne at six o'clock in the morning. The last of the party people had gone home. We'd swept the floor. It was almost bright again outside. You could see the light changing in the sky above Mughal's Newsagents and the Aberdeen Angus Steak House.

—We've done it. Us. We've come through the whole

thing and we've done it on our own with no one's help only our own.

One of us said it. Both of us meant it. We were a couple. I thought we were the perfect couple. All right, being the perfect couple was part of the contract with the brewery but I thought we really were. We were there for everyone who doubted there really was love and connection. We laid our good days and our bad days out on the counter and let them see how we always managed to win on points.

Maybe some days we thought we pushed too hard. Maybe the odd time we wished so much of our contact wasn't a pooling together of strength to drive through the challenges exhaustion would have made us avoid on our own. But when we thought and wished that we thought and wished together. And together we knew that in ten years there would be days of relative rest. There would be a soft green couch. A timeshare. And bank statements casually left lying for weeks on a big table in a long hall.

In Rathbawn Cathedral, I ran my tongue around the roof of my mouth. Trying to forget where I was and remember a taste. The taste of love.

It tasted something like vinegar. The vinegar which gave the tang to the top of the lamb kebabs we would take away from the Greek restaurant at that time in the morning when all the stools had been turned upside down and stacked in heaps by the walls of the King William.

We went there first when the snow was inches deep and we couldn't face the trek to the Octopuses Garden Fish Bar.

The manager brought us two glasses of sambuca, set the spirit alight and laughed at our amazement. He brought those glasses down to us many nights. Lydia's eyes would follow the sambuca flame like a child's looking at a sparkler.

He introduced us to his friends, old Greek and Cypriot men who kept their coats on and sat at tables pulled up tight

75

to the counter. They read Greek newspapers and slowly ate olives off side-plates.

—You are good people, you are good people.

He often said that as we went out into the night. I suppose we were.

I stayed in London in my head. It was the day me and Lydia bought the tape-recorder. The first thing we bought together. The first week we went out together. We walked into an electrical shop on the Walworth Road and I set off the loudest alarm I'd ever heard by touching one of the models on display. A thick industrial-looking black yoke.

Nothing would do Lydia except to get this dinky double-deck job. White with pink buttons. Very chi-chi. We bought a few tapes at East Street market on our way back to the Flock of Swans. In celebration. None of the tapes were what it said on the case. But that was immaterial. One of the bands was called 'It's Immaterial'.

Only there was this one song on one tape. So relaxed at the beginning it sounded like it wasn't sure if it should start or not. Then the voice came through. Bob Marley. Relaxed in love. Cocooned inside the belief there was definitely such a thing.

> *Stir it up little darling*
> *Stir it up come on baby*
> *Come on and stir it up little darling*
> *Stir it up oh*
> *It's been a long long time*
> *Since I got you on my mind*
> *And now you are here*
> *I said it's so clear*
> *To see what we can do*
> *Just me and you*
> *Come on and stir it up little darling*
> *Stir it up little darling.*

I looked at Lydia. Lydia looked at me. She asked me the name of the tape. I looked at the cover.

—'Kaya'. It's called 'Kaya'.

'Kaya'. Bob Marley. And the Wailers. Fair play to the Marley buck. And his Wailers. He was dead. Lydia was dead. I hadn't played the tape since she died. No way. Couldn't do it. It was only a song. But everything is only something. When Lydia was alive I played the song six times every day. I hoped the woman Bob wrote it for listened to him.

The tape wasn't called 'Kaya' at all. But that made our daughter's name seem all the more chosen.

Poor oul Bob was dead too. It was all death these days. Standing there in the Cathedral carpark after the removal I knew that the revenge was still with me. For Johnny and Lydia and Bob. I'd not been able to get any revenge for Lydia. Except on myself. On Vinnie to a lesser degree. And Kerrie to a greater. But there had to be some revenge handy in Rathbawn. For Johnny. And Lydia. And Bob.

Not that I was sure what revenge was except that it had to do with violence. With a lot of violence. I hadn't drawn a belt on anyone in years. It seemed a silly idea. I didn't even know how to start getting this revenge. But I did know I would get some. Some satisfaction. It was my town too and before I left it I wanted to feel like a man and not a pinky-faced gossan who gets boxed on the lug and made stand in a corner. I wanted that at least. Kaya pulled the hem of my jacket.

—Can we go home, Dad? I'm tired and I'm really hungry.

Kaya was outside this. She had her mother's eyes but I wasn't sure if I'd been looking straight into them. I needed some justice.

0800's voice boomed round the house from the sitting-room and told people the difference between the Druze, the Christian Militia and the Hezbollah.

Eddie Clyne was rinsing glasses in the kitchen. He picked up a crate of Guinness and winked at me.

—Joe Donoghue came up with this. Come on into the living-room. Johnny would knock great oul enjoyment out of a wake.

—He would if some other fucker was dead.

Oul Kenny Gorman crucified the fuck out of Red River Valley in the sitting-room. No one listened but they gave him a great roar and a cheer when he finished in case he tried to sing a second song.

A tall, tall woman with curly auburn hair perched on the side of a chair in front of the fire. Eddie plonked the crate of Guinness on the floor and himself in the chair. He slipped his hand into the long, tall woman's hand. She looked over at me. I looked at how those legs were set off by the extended belt soldered on to her hips.

—Paul, this is my wife, Sonia.

—Jesus.

I said it before a more appropriate response came to mind. The last time I'd seen Sonia Dunbar she'd been in her confirmation outfit.

—Nice to meet you. It's awful about Johnny.

Sonia sounded like she meant both sentences.

—Elle the Body.

Beetlejuice spoke from the corner of the room where he was looking at the framed Papal Marriage Blessing Mam still kept on the wall for some reason.

—Elle the Body herself.

He said it again. Sonia Dunbar's voice emerged as a coo.

—It is nice to meet you.

Eddie looked at his feet but there was a sort of a glowing Ready Brek kid set to him. Beetlejuice mucked around with the dial of the radio. Midland Radio came on.

—This is *The Leuuve Zone* with Jamie Knox.

Jamie Knox tried to stretch his accent on a rack and give

it the flavour of an American city where the docks would be called the Bay Area.

—That fuckdog is from Cavan.

—How do you know, Beetlejuice?

—I robbed his house once.

The Leuuve Zone was on the last legs when I said I was hitting the hay. The reel in my head hadn't to do with the drink. Or the dope. Not completely. I'd lost my rhythm since I landed in Rathbawn. Things seemed to be happening to me. As if me being back caused a change.

Maybe it was the dope after all.

I couldn't get to sleep in my bedroom that had been mine and Johnny's bedroom and then Johnny's bedroom. I couldn't do anything. I just sat on the bed and put my hands over the eyes. I didn't even unloosen my tie. Green-and-red paisleys. Lydia. That row over my making a mess of the roster so she had to work a busy Saturday night when she was eight months gone with Kaya. Ties to settle arguments. Family ties.

I thought about the day. About Beetlejuice, about Dalton Dunbar's way of rolling a spliff, about how Sonia Dunbar that was looked.

It was always the same. I was thinking about how to describe my day to Lydia. But then I realized I didn't need to find the words. Because Lydia was not there. And it didn't matter to her what I thought. Because she would never think anything again.

I flipped open the door of the locker beside the bed. What did I expect to find? Maybe a little black Letts diary with its own pencil tucked into the spine. 'My year' by Johnny Kelly. Important dates. Today I am going to be murdered. And he would have underlined the name of his murderer. Which would be printed in neat block-capital, application-form letters.

No diary. The only object in the locker was a football

programme with a big colour cover on it. From that European game Rathbawn Rovers had two years ago. They got stuffed by some Belgian mob. The only time I'd ever seen the name Rathbawn on the BBC. On *Sportsnight* in the European football results. I did get a bit of a twinge when I saw it.

The match programme was all in whatever language they speak in Belgium.

—*Het lot koppelde* club *voor de eerste ronde aan de* Rovers *uit her Ierse* Rathbawn, *een mooie* warming-up *voor het grote werk.*

You couldn't argue with that. Mam said Johnny was over to Europe a good few times. I asked her what he was working at in town.

—I'm not 100 per cent sure but I think it was something in the security line. Himself and that young Reilly lad had a security firm, I think.

I got a bit of a laugh out of it first. The thought of someone hiring one of the Reillys to do security for them. Rob All Security. Pull the other one and it plays a hornpipe and sells raffle tickets as well. Still. You don't know. You can't know anything about people really. I knew nothing about my brother Johnny because I'd been away for eight years. And even if I'd lived in the same house as him for every day of those eight years there was still a fairly sound argument that said I'd know next to fuck-all about him.

—Hi, trouble's here.

Sonia Clyne. Sonia Dunbar that was. Elle the Body. Whoever she was she'd walked into the room without knocking.

She was model-beautiful. You see that sometimes. Beauty in strange places. Like a folly in the bog. Sonia talked about Johnny.

—A lot of people misses him. Do you miss him, Paul?

—Of course I do. He was the only brother I had.

—Suppose. He was something else. Everyone was mad about him. You always knew he was there. It's a sort of a thing that now you can see the gap in the place he should be.

She hung her head to one side. Her make-up had an orange tint. I tried to look deep underneath it but there wasn't the hint of a bump or a crease there. She smelt of some expensive perfume. I'd smelt Lydia's wrists often enough at sample counters to know what the expensive stuff smelt like. Lydia's left wrist had a small brown mole resting at the start of the longest visible vein in her arm. Sonia's hands sat in her lap. Her wedding ring seemed to catch the flickering light of the bulb over our heads.

—I must change that oul bulb. I think it's burning through the holder as well.

—Poor Johnny. He was always a good friend to me. He always understood me.

Sonia gave off a whimper and flung her arms round my neck. Her chin rested on my shoulder. There was a sharp bone there that dug into me. I didn't move away because of that. I moved away because I was scared. She turned her back on me and stooped to rearrange her hair in the dressing-table mirror. Her breath came in those long, juddering gasps that Johnny's had when he had his worst asthma attacks. In this room.

—I'm so unhappy. I'm so fucking unhappy.

Then she gulped and her face changed back to the shiny happy one she'd brought into the room.

—Paul. Has my mascara run?

—No. I don't think so.

—Good. Yer one in Plunkett's told me it was waterproof but I didn't believe her. You know, you're not like your brother at all, at all.

—Come on, me oul flower, we'll go down to the sitting-room. Eddie'll think I've murdered you.

She lit up a white fag. It doused the air with a sickly smell of singed Silvermints.

—Eddie? Eddie thinks I'm gone home. I told him I was going an hour ago.

I twigged what the word sashay meant as she did that out the bedroom door and into the hall and left me trying out a foolish treacherous laugh as the door closed quietly.

Still no sleep. I looked at the clock. Three forty-seven. I switched on Midland Radio to kill the silence.

> *Twenty-four hours of music every day,*
> *It helps you keep the blues away.*

Jingle balls. It was twenty-four hours because they switched on the CD player before they knocked off for the night. Then the CD player would go and banjax itself and keep repeating the first lines of a song over and over again:

> *I'll try to love again,*
> *Trytrytrytrytrytrytrytrytrytrytrytrytrytrytrytrytrytry.*

I switched it back on at half four. Same thing. Bastards.

—Trytrytrytrytrytrytrytrytrytrytrytrytrytrytrytrytrytry.

I went for a slash. Tracey came out of the jacks just before I touched the door handle. Still in her good removal clobber.

—What's going on, head? Is there still a gang down there?

—There's no gang down there, only me. Somebody has to clean the mess up, you know. It's a pity I'm the only one who thinks of other people.

—Uuum. Yeah. Why do they call Eddie Clyne's wife Elle the Body?

—'Cause if we called her what she should be called, she'd have us up the steps to the courthouse.

I switched the radio on again when I got back into bed.

—Trytrytrytrytrytrytrytrytrytrytrytrtytrytrytry.

Click. Zonk.

Five

Please be Good, You Know You Should

I woke up in the morning, thanked the stars I was alive. I did really. Always a big bonus, starting the day alive. After what you worry about when you're trying to slope off to the Land of Nod.

If I should die before I wake.

A point in favour of drink. If you've a gang of gargle in you the hay can be hit without wondering if tonight is the night you're going to snuff it. Off you go into uncomplicated sleep and dreams about entering a cheese-tasting competition with Cindy Crawford or enjoying a life in Provence with the sexy bunny from the Cadbury's Caramel ad.

Jar can wipe out everything if you have enough of it. You could get killed on the way home and you wouldn't twig it if you were pissed enough. There you'd be pottering around the next day wondering about your jolly japes of the night previous. Where was I? What did I do? How did I get home?

Then about six in the evening it'd come to you. Shit, I was murdered last night. And straight down you'd drop. Stone-dead. The realization would kill you. Like Wile E. Coyote when he goes over the cliff and he's running on thin air. Sound till he looks down and tries to plant his feet.

Twilight Zone. Dananana dananana dananana.

I travelled to the Cathedral for the funeral service with Francie and Liz. Young Jennifer sang a song to herself. Repeating the same sounds. Half breath, half song.

—Shuhsoshuh, shuhsoshuh, shuhsoshuh.

—Jennifer's full of beans this morning, said Francie.

He opened the back door to let Liz and the kids clamber out into the Cathedral carpark.

—The more you fart the better you feel, so eat beans with every meal, said Jennifer.

—Don't be disgusting, you.

Liz tried to look angry but it was the first time I'd seen her smile in eight years.

It was five to eleven when I noticed Mam wasn't in the church. She should have been in the front seats but I walked down to the porch in case she was chatting to some of her cronies there. Not a sign of her.

Up and down the aisle again in case I hadn't been looking properly. No. No Mam. Another scan of the Cathedral. Mam definitely not to be had. This was daft.

0800 and Francie each thought she'd come to the church in the other's car. Tracey copped what was up and made frantic signals at 0800.

—I better go and see is she back in the house.

Jesus wept, what a palaver.

The priest was making his way on to the altar when 0800 and Mam arrived. Mam piled up the aisle at such a clip 0800 had to break into a quick march to keep up. You could tell

86

she'd been out in the rain. Water cascaded off her as she knelt.

—Praise to you, Lord Jesus Christ.

I always wondered what Imprimi Potest and Nihil Obstat were. They sounded like Czechoslovakian teams who got knocked out in the second round of the European Cup Winners Cup.

The priest was one of those performing fuckers. The deep voice. The meaningful pause. And the come-to-me-all-who-labour hand gestures. I wondered if he got tired having to do his old hits all the time. He might feel like throwing in a few bits of the Koran or the Buddha book. Just to be on the safe side. In case he'd backed the wrong horse.

Muldoon, that was it, Father Muldoon.

—Johnny Kelly was one of a well-known local family. His family have always been regular mass-goers and I know personally that his mother is a woman of great faith. Nuala —

Pause for a soulful look over at Mam. Little did he know that only for 0800 he would have had to go out to the front door if he wanted to do that.

—That faith will help you overcome the grief you are feeling at the tragic death of your son. None of us are saints and Johnny was no exception. He had his faults no more than the rest of us. But he was a cheerful and popular young man known for his generosity to his friends and his interest in other members of the community. The old saying goes, 'If you want to know me, come and live with me,' and Johnny's true character is best reflected by the dedication he showed to his mother at home. Johnny Kelly's very real love for his mother is an example to us all in these days when it is trendy to criticize the family unit. Johnny Kelly may not have been an outwardly religious young man but, in his own way, he had great faith. We all must have faith at this very traumatic time.

Where do they get them from? Some sort of a sermon-preaching course in Maynooth? With FAS running it. Or maybe there's a big blue book filled with sermons for all occasions. *The Encyclopedia Sermonica*. There might be a lad who lives in a big castle on top of a hill in Wicklow. He reads all the death notices every morning, makes a few phone calls and faxes out the personalized orations to the Presbytery in the afternoon.

Orations. Great word. Remember your history. It's like garlic, it will repeat whether you want it to or not.

—And while Ireland holds these graves, Ireland unfree shall never be at peace.

Revenge again. The funeral antidote. It's all you can count on.

Father Muldoon was in full spate now. Playing a blinder. Someone way down the Cathedral coughed. One of those raspy, splattery coughs that come out when you're trying to clear your throat and keep the noise down at the same time.

—Because, and let's make no mistake about it, death is the one certainty in our lives. It is what we all have in common. We all must die. We know that. The sentence of our life is already written. We can embellish it. We can alter the letters. But it is death which inserts the full stop and we have no say in that.

Where do they get them from?

I let his voice pass through my head and looked at one of the altar-girls. It was all altar-girls these days. She knelt at the back of the altar. On both knees. She changed to her left. After about a minute she bowed her lips into a silent

—Ooooow.

She switched to her right knee. Then executed the whole sequence in reverse. She clasped her hands and decided to examine them, waggling them in front of her face before looking pleadingly up at the roof.

—Death can come at any time and it is up to us, as good Christians, to always be prepared for it.

The little altar-girl hit the server beside her a puck into the ribs and told her a joke. The other girl looked away sombrely so she had to go back to waggling her fingers.

> *Dying, you destroyed our death.*
> *Rising, you restored our life.*
> *Lord Jesus, come in glory.*

The priest's voice boomed around the shop. So did the voices of the folk choir. Fuck me backwards. A woodwork teacher from the college leading the way on guitar. If I'd wanted the Mamas and the Papas playing at my brother's funeral I'd have booked them myself. There was something to be said for the oul Faith of Our Fathers all the same. But I couldn't think what it was.

I was nearly on my way over to the car when I remembered what was left to be done. Twitch the shoulder. Think of how strong you are. And how they do it on all those IRA funerals you see on the telly.

Lydia had been cremated. Her ashes were in an urn. On a mantelpiece. In Govan. It was another thing I would not be able to tell Mam. Or any of the family. It seemed right then. But strange now. Now that me and Uncle Jimmy and Uncle Gerry and Uncle Tony were at one corner each of this wooden container. Traipsing along behind the hearse. Like Joseph's young buck hitting the road to Golgotha. My left ear chafed against the side of the coffin. I still hoped it might hear whispering.

—Get a move on, Paul. I'm not dead at all, you know. Wait till ye've carted me all the way out to Templekeeran and I'll make a buck-lep out of this coffin and show ye there's been a mistake. It is a mistake, Paul.

When we were through the gates and walking towards the cluster of Kelly graves. I knew I'd make it. See what you can do when you really put your mind to it. Little victories. But big efforts to win them. 0800 made an expansive circling motion with his hand.

—A couple of days of Israeli shell-fire on South Lebanon would fill this place.

—Would you ever be quiet.

Tracey lunged forward and pressed both of her hands against my right palm. Her face couldn't show sadness but tears dropped metronomically.

—Oh, Paul. Oh, Paul.

I caught her in my arms. Her kids looked frightened. 0800 shifted his weight from one foot to the other like he wanted to scratch himself.

Jesus, we're all so useless sometimes.

Uncle Jimmy spoke for the first time when the last wreath landed beside the headstone.

—The man that's down there wouldn't have much time for all this shite.

Plastic boxes. Wooden boxes. A Players Navy Cut box poked out of the pocket of Mattie Beadle's trousers as he methodically emptied his shovel with the casualness of Kaya shaking clinging sugar off a wet teaspoon.

Tracey had recovered by the time we walked away from the grave and left Martin Joyce and Mattie Beadle at the job they were used to. From the gates I saw them both light cigarettes. Cupping the matches in their hands to defeat the wind that blew in that wide-open scrap of land no matter what the weather was like in the rest of Rathbawn. Tracey whispered to me as we walked towards the cars.

—She thought ye were coming back to collect her and bring her to the Cathedral. I had a feeling ye were gone but no way would she let us take her. She said ye were going to bring her. Kevin found her walking down.

Mam was in the front seat of Francie's car. I felt like a kid in the back seat. Stupid to lose your licence. Stupider again to drive when you had it lost and get bagged a second time and banned for a few more years. I suppose I'd got the few pound for the car at least. Mam started on Liz before Francie started the engine.

—How could ye leave me to walk to my own son's funeral? Didn't ye know I was going to the Cathedral with ye?

—Mammy, didn't you know we were gone?

—Didn't ye know I was going to the Cathedral with ye? I went with ye yesterday. Did it not make sense to have the same arrangements today?

—Mammy, but we thought . . .

—You know what thought did, Liz. Hadn't ye a right at least to tell Tracey and Kevin ye weren't coming back? I could have waited there till after eleven. I nearly did, fool that I am.

Liz didn't bother interrupting again. She just looked out the window and toyed nervously with Jennifer's hair. Francie kept his eyes tunnel-vision-straight on the road. His knuckles whitened occasionally on the steering wheel. Kaya broke the silence.

—What did thought do, Dad?

—He stuck a feather in the ground and thought it'd grow a hen.

Francie stopped the car outside Donoghue's. Mam stayed in her seat when he opened the passenger door.

—Take me home, Francie. I don't want to go in there. I'll be all right in the house on my own.

—Ah, Missus Kelly, come on in.

—I wouldn't be able to have a drink this early in the day. Ye go ahead, I'll take something and go asleep for a few hours. I'm very tired.

Francie stood resting his hand at the top of the door. The

kids were already at the door of Donoghue's. The noise of a packed pub came out to us. Liz was frozen on the footpath. She glanced over at me.

—Fuck you, Mam, come in. It's not often the whole family is together. The girls'll go down to the house with you after a bit.

—I wouldn't be up to it, Paul.

—Come on, Mam. For the sake of the rest of us.

—I'll come in for one but I won't enjoy it.

Shadowy fragments of conversation had carried a long way on the Templekeeran cross-winds.

—A few people not here.

—Hard to blame them.

—Nothing against the family.

But the more I thought about them the less sure I was of what I heard. The disparate mumble in graveyards can sound like anything you want to hear.

I was getting there again by four o'clock. So were half the Park. The other half and Liz and Tracey went back to the house with Mam.

Elle the Body was leaving the Ladies as I quit the Gents. The sweet aura of female drunkenness scented her breath. She was stocious. Her right arm looped around my shoulder.

—How are you? How are you now?

—OK, Sonia. Still sad though.

—This fucking pub. It's a kip, right. The light is gone in the ladies' so you can't see what you're fucking doing. I bet I'm all over the place, am I?

Her hair was falling over her face but she was still perfectly sewn into the black dress she wore to the funeral. I told her she looked 100 per cent apart from the bra strap which had fallen well below her tanned right shoulder.

—Aw, yeah, I see. My arm is all sore. You couldn't put the yoke back in place, could you?

—What about your other arm?

—Go on. You can say that arm is banjaxed too. I might have pins and needles in it.

The door from the bar opened. We both jumped. Young Robbie stalked through in his most self-conscious-man manner and proudly kicked the gents' door open. I wanted to make a joke. But I couldn't think of a joke. Not even a bad one. So I closed my fingers on the thin string of her bra strap and slid it gently up to her shoulder. My hand brushed against the flesh there. It was cool like something that had been kept in a freezer. The coolness floated somewhere above the heat of Donoghue's.

—Thanks.

—Don't mention it.

—I better go in. My honey is inside. See you later, alligator.

Robbie came out of the jacks and danced around me with his hands held high in front of his face.

—Put your guard up, Uncle Paul, I'm going starting boxing soon.

I walked back into the bar. Sometimes you just can't be bothered.

Francie and 0800 sat together at the counter talking to Joe Donoghue. I joined them. Joe shoved a pint of Guinness in front of me. I flung a fiver on the counter. 0800 smoothed it out before he handed it back to me.

—Joe's getting these.

—Thanks, Joe.

—For nothing, boys. For nothing.

—Good fucking men. You know, we're good fucking men, the three of us. Three decent men that never done any harm to nobody, just having pints and minding our own fucking business.

It was one of Francie's longest ever speeches. His head dropped as if he was going to fall asleep. He lifted it again and put his arms around us.

—We know what it's all about, Joe. Me and my two friends. Lunatics is what we are. And good fucking men.

0800 laughed.

—Good fucking men.

Three pint glasses clinked together. We were looking at ourselves from the outside at that moment. Brothers-in-law. Rivalry, jealousy and secrecy all cheerfully mingled. 0800 told Joe to take a bottle of brandy down from the optic.

—This man here, Joe, is my friend, my good friend. And this buck – are you listening to me, Joe? – is my young brother-in-law that was only a gossan when I saw him last. This buck, and he's a good lad, Joe, the brother of my wife that I love, Joe, you know, and some people might say she orders me about but there's not many around like her. Boys, my mates, we'll drink a toast to the family.

He poured three double brandies.

—You see, in other countries there's no optics, you see, they measure it with the eye and pour it out by the hand. By the hand. Ye'd know about these things, you see, if ye were ever in foreign countries. You see, if ye were in the army, I'm in the army you see and no one'll ever make a laugh out of it to my face whatever they might think. Corporal Kevin McGoey of the Cavalry Squadron and proud of it. Foreign travel, you see, it's good for the knowledge side of things. Ye were nowhere – well, I know you were in England, Paul, but England's not foreign. England is only Ireland with cunts living in it.

We banged the glasses on the counter and drank the brandy down in one gulp.

—*Aris* Anthony.

I suppose we were all looking for a way out after the second repeat performance. Francie had the good sense to give it to us.

—I suppose we better go and talk to the people.

—If you're not up to it . . .

—I didn't say that.

—Ah, come on, 0800, he's right.

—He is. I was only pulling his chain.

—It'd be a change from pulling your own one.

Eddie Clyne wasn't drinking. He was sitting at a table where you could see occasional glimpses of the wood through a forest of pint glasses. A half-full glass of flat Ballygowan was sitting in front of him and a half-empty bottle of the stuff beside him.

—You're sure you won't have a drink, Eddie?

—No. No. I'm grand. If I went back on the beer, I'd be scared I'd go on a mad batter.

—You're sure now?

—Oh, yeah. This stuff does me grand. I'll be driving home anyways. One of us has to be sober in my house.

—Dalton Dunbar came over.

—Hit that cunt a box if he's bothering you. It's the only language he understands. Are you on for going up to the Dandy Diner, Mary Colreavy's hen party is on but we're all invited.

I was going to say I couldn't because it was the night of my brother's funeral but I didn't. I didn't have any place else I wanted to go and I couldn't face going back to the house. Not yet at least. So I went and left 0800 and Francie at the bar together.

A squad slowed down and drove along beside us for a few yards when we left Donoghue's. It was pulling away when Beetlejuice let a wolf-whistle at it. The car reversed and Cosgrave stuck his head out the window.

—Does someone have a problem?

—You what?

—You'll whistle soon enough if you're brought down to the barracks. You'd need to watch yourselves.

—You must be fucking hearing things, guard. First sign of madness, that.

The cop slammed the door. A dozen whistles in different keys started up the second it closed. A couple of cans clattered against the back of the squad as it sped away.

The Dandy Diner must have been cursed at one stage by someone who knew how to curse. A Nevin or a McDonagh. Whoever owned it always put a ridiculous name on it. Once it had been the Nashville Rooms. Another time Kades Kounty. At one stage it was even Nijinsky's Nite Spot. That name would have delighted the Gay Swimming Club who came into the King William every Thursday night for a few pints after leaving the Lido.

A space opened up in front of us when we walked in. It developed into a funnel which fed us straight through to the bar even though the joint was wedged. Two of a Kind were playing. I got jammed against a pillar. A poster threatened to fall on my head.

OKEY DOKEY KARAOKE. EVERY MONDAY NIGHT WITH P.J. AND MARGARET. SUBSTANTIAL CASH PRIZES.

The hen party sat in one corner of the pub with their chairs drawn round in a circle. Mary Colreavy in the middle had a party hat on her head and streamers waterfalling from her shoulders. I wondered if Lydia's hen had been like this. It struck me I'd never asked her about it.

Clinger arrived and hovered over my shoulder. He reached to shake hands with me.

—All right.

—All right. I'll buy you a pint. I reckoned you must be broke when you didn't show up in Donoghue's.

He winked at me and extended his leg so it touched the pillar. Then he reached towards his shoe.

—I have a few pound put away, see. And if we'd gone to Donoghue's the quare one would have known I had it and I'd have to give her some.

Clinger took off his shoe and reached into a blue sock that

covered all of his left foot except for the big toe that poked out of a frayed hole and wriggled around frantically like it was trying to dig into sand as the tide went out. A black circle covered the top end of the nail.

—The oul sock, you see, it's the only safe place in the end.

He took out two tenners and brushed some flakes of skin off their surface. I still bought the first round. We talked about football.

I bought the next round as well. And put on a chaser for myself. Beetlejuice was there when I got back from the bar. His hands shook a lot. He lifted his pint to his mouth and left it down a couple of times without taking more than a sup. When he spoke his lips shook too.

—I'm nervous, Paul, I just am. I have this feeling and it's the same feeling I had the night Johnny was killed. I know something's going happening.

Beetlejuice stuttered through most of the words. He reached his hand out for his pint and pulled it back before it got there.

—That fuck. That fuck, him, he's up to something.

An old man loitered at the bottom of the stairs. He was hopping a thick brown walking stick off the floor. The pub was at basting temperature but he was rigged out in a thick pair of specs, a tweed cap and a long coat buttoned to the top.

—He's at something. I'll skull him.

—He's a fucking oul man. What could he be at?

—I'm going to fucking skull him.

Beetlejuice got to within a couple of yards of the old geezer before Richie Fee caught him. They had a few words. Beetlejuice had stopped shaking when he came back.

—Richie told me the score, boys. It's all copacetic. Jesus, such crack, wait till you see it.

A couple of the hens walked up to the stage. Two of a Kind launched straight away into an instrumental. The one they play on telly at the end of the World Snooker Championship when they show the funny shots. A big movement from our side of the pub over to the chair where Mary Colreavy was. Beetlejuice pulled my arm.

—Come over. The crack is going starting.

The band started to run through the tune a second time. People were standing on chairs now and looking into the circle of hens. It reminded me of the time in the Horse and Groom a squaddie bet he'd be able to drink a pint of sick.

—Wait till you see this for crack.

Beetlejuice was happy. The band looked down the pub like they were waiting for some sort of signal. The pub went silent as the old man dondered towards Mary Colreavy. He leaned heavily on his stick. I half expected him to drop before he got to her. He peered at her through his double-glazed glasses.

—Are you the girleen who's getting married? Sure you'll give us a biteen of an oul kiss.

His lips puckered out about half a mile in front of his face. Mary looked around for some assistance but there wasn't any. Belinda Greer was breaking her heart laughing. Beetlejuice snickered. The old guy put his arm around Mary's neck and planted a big slimy kiss on her lips before jumping into the air and clicking his heels together. He threw the tweed cap on the floor.

—*Hasta la vista*, baby.

The glasses, the coat, the cap and the stick were all on the floor within ten seconds of that spake and the old geezer was now a young guy with muscles on him that looked like they were going to burst. All he had on was a deep suntan and a pair of boxer shorts. A noise sprinted round the pub.

—Woooo.

Even the barmen stopped what they were doing and looked over at the ex-old man sitting on Mary's knee. Belinda bent double with laughing. Mary looked terrified.

Her new pal planted another kiss on her lips and got a roar from the hens as he flexed the muscles on his arm. They shone under the lights. He looked like a chicken covered in cooking oil.

—A lot of them bucks is queer, said someone a couple of yards behind me.

It was a man's voice. Not one of the women had touched a drink since bucko shed his coat and fifty years. Missus Fee looked like one of those Charismatics who have just been possessed by the Spirit of the Lord. But she wasn't speaking in tongues.

—You're lovely, you're lovely. Go on and show us what you've got.

The stripper jumped off Mary's lap and gave a little bow before pulling a string which disintegrated his boxers into a heap on the floor. For a second everyone thought he didn't have anything at all on. His arse was bare. But there was a little string running around the front and an orange pouch for him to cram his tackle into. He bent down to his coat and took out a piece of paper. The chest muscles got another flex before he started declaiming.

> *Hello Mary here I am*
> *Your saucy sexy stripogram*
> *Please be good you know you should*
> *Let's get on this could be good*
> *I've got a present I thought would suit*
> *Now I want you to suck my . . .*

He paused. A couple of people bellowed:
—Flute.
He waited a couple more seconds before he took the banana out of his coat.
—Fruit.
—You've some fucking body on you.

A woman's shout from the balcony. I held my breath and tried to hold in my stomach. I wouldn't say I was the only one imagining what I'd look like in front of a pub of women with my kit off. You could jog, I suppose. And there's American exercises that get you in shape in just ten minutes a day and you end up only having to do them three times a week. You could go on the Scarsdale Diet. Fuck it. He probably wasn't happy in his life.

Belinda got hold of him by the pouch. His lad popped out but he just grinned and flicked it expertly back in with his left hand. All the men were disappointed it was a good size. He arranged the banana so it protruded from his pouch.

—Suction. It must be, said a voice full of awe.

The women clattered the tables. The stripper pushed Mary's head towards his groin. She shied her head away at first. The buck she was marrying was in the army with 0800. He'd been going out with Mary for six years and he bursted anyone who looked crooked at her. I was fierce sorry he wasn't in the Dandy Diner. Someone should have asked him to come along.

A drum-roll from Two of a Kind. Snap. Mary's head came up. She had the top half of the banana in her mouth. A dozen flashes went off at once and the stripper threw on his coat and got the fuck out of there. He was just past the table when Missus Fee got him a pinch on the arse you could nearly feel just from seeing it. Another woman grabbed him by the kecks and tried to yank them off. He bolted for the door with a gang of women after him. Screaming. I'd never heard screaming like it. He nearly knocked down the barman who was bringing down a cake in the shape of a muscle-man.

Someone grabbed me around the waist and the next thing I knew I was in a circle twirling around the floor with Two of a Kind playing the can-can and of course there's always one header who levers himself up on his neighbour's shoulders and does a wild kick with both of his feet up in the air and falls down then and nearly brings everyone else with them and it was Beetlejuice naturally enough. He was gone fucking hyper.

Mary opened a package. Belinda helped her. They removed the wrapping and took out a pair of big Y-fronty knickers about the size of two wigwams.

—Woooo.

The Jordan woman who used be a midwife crammed a big slice of the muscle-man cake into her mouth. Oozy black cherries dangled from it. She picked them off and put them into the ashtray. A few of Mary's buddies stood her up and put her legs into the knickers. Belinda planted a kiss that left a ruby smear of lipstick on Mary's face.

The can-can stopped and myself and Missus Fee were left leaning awkwardly against each other and trying to remember what the weather had been like so we could talk about it.

Two of a Kind played a Country song about honky-tonks and broken hearts. Beetlejuice hugged Mary Colreavy. He was enjoying himself like . . . No. Like nothing. You think of these things later. More significance. More Columbo. He stuck his legs into the giant underpants. First the left. Then the right. He put his arms around Mary and they danced. Suspended in their giant nappy with green balloons flying over their heads. Myself, Clinger and Dalton stood in a circle and headed a balloon to each other. Each determined not to be the first to let it hit the ground or float away.

—Fuck's sake. Another one of these lads, they're gone mad on them altogether.

Clinger controlled the balloon with his shoulder.

—Handball.

Myself and Dalton at the same time. The guitarist in Two of a Kind did one of those long, twiddly-bit, Jesus-I'm-Eddie-Van-Halen-can't-you-nearly-see-the-smoke-rising-off-me-fingers solos. I couldn't make out what the song was because he was gone so much to town on it.

—What's that song, boys?

—Jesus. It's a bit much now all the same, a second lad, it nearly knocks the good out of it.

—What? I didn't catch you right.

—One of those stripogram bucks again.

—What's the name of that song?

A tall man in a long black coat, wearing a plastic gorilla false face topped by a baseball cap, pushed his way through the crowd. A dancing arm clipped the side of his head and knocked his cap skew-ways. He stopped and straightened it very deliberately with his left hand. Then he patted the cap down on his nut to make sure it was properly balanced. With his left hand again. He held his right arm under his coat like it was broken and suspended in a sling. The cap was a Utah Jazz one. You had to laugh at this grinning gorilla face making its way across the pub. People smiled and stood back to let him through.

—Beetlejuice. Beetlejuice Reilly. Noelie Reilly.

The voice came from underneath the mask. Beetlejuice and Mary were still jumping up and down.

—Beetlejuice Reilly. Is that you?

Beetlejuice tried to turn round. The upper half of his body swivelled but his legs stayed facing Mary Colreavy.

—Away we go, said the false face.

A revolver came out from under the coat. Beetlejuice's gob was fixed in a toothy smile when the gun blew it away. He staggered and the man stepped forward and shot him in the back of the head. A tiny burst of flame seemed to jump from the gun. The gorilla's hand was rock-steady.

Mary Colreavy's face was covered in blood and goo. She screeched as Beetlejuice fell and dragged her to the floor. Both of them were still trapped in those monster Y-fronts. Nothing was left of Beetlejuice's head only a sight of blood. Mary was in hysterics. Two of a Kind stopped playing. The singer crouched down behind one of the amps. People knocked over tables and chairs as they tried to get out of the pub.

Beetlejuice wasn't moving. Mary kicked like mad to try and disentangle herself from him. Belinda shoved through the crowd and bent down to her. The gunman aimed carefully and put a third shot through Beetlejuice's head. I heard the sound of something soggy falling on a concrete path from a great height. Beetlejuice's body jerked. Mary's body had to make the same movement. She was gone pure white in the face. She looked past Belinda who had pulled her head off the floor and was cradling her.

Mary's face and neck and the front of her little black dress were all covered with whatever comes out when someone's head explodes. She slipped out of Belinda's arms and lay on the floor again. Blood seeped out of what used to be Beetlejuice.

—What's my name, what's my name.

The gunman's words were all muffled by the plastic mask. He turned and walked towards the door like he didn't give a breeze. I tried to shrink back into one of the alcoves. I had a feeling he'd want to shoot me if he knew I was in the pub. Clinger and Dalton started after him.

—Get the cunt. Stop him.

Have-a-go heroes. He turned and fired a couple of shots at them. They seemed like noisier shots. The Dandy Diner filled up with the sound of firecrackers let off in a small space. Clinger was on the ground with blood soaking through his shirt. Dalton was plugged in the arm. The gunman did a little dance.

—How you like me now, motherfuckers. How you like me now.

It was a fake American accent but it wouldn't have fooled anyone except maybe for one of those women who refused to believe that Big Tex and the Rangers were a gang of lads from Sheepwalk who worked in the abattoir. He let off a couple more shots but his hand was jumping around now. A hole appeared in one of the windows. Glasses tinkled. He walked out the side door of the Dandy Diner.

A car revved up and took off. It left two perky blasts of a horn behind it in the night air. The killer had been wearing those Converse basketball boots with the star at the side of them. It's funny what you think of. I couldn't take in much else.

Mary lay stock-still in a corner with a gang of her friends screaming at everybody to do something. Clinger had dragged himself up on to a chair. He leaned back with his shirt open and blood slowly trickling down in different streams. Richie Fee walked Dalton out the door. Dalton's arm hung down like it wasn't really attached to him.

Blood all over the gaff. Little specks in the ashtrays. Splotches on the walls. Long streaks on the glass of the alcoves. Spots of it soaked through the cheap paper Dandy Diner beer mats. The late Noel Reilly lay face down in a big pool of the stuff with the woman of the Jordans who'd been a midwife hunkered down beside him. She shook her head.

I was left on my own in my alcove when everyone else moved on to the street. There I was, looking at what was left of Beetlejuice lying there like an old Guy Fawkes fucked into an estate lift in the middle of November. Rag and bone. Stupid bastard. Friend of my brother. The late John Kelly. Whatever the fuck the story was, someone had it in for them big time.

The light show outside. Ambulances and squads and the streetlamps. And the noise of the sirens adding to it. Except you couldn't hardly hear them. You could hear the crying in the street a bit better. But what you could hear most was the screaming of the women. It kept at the same pitch and level until they sounded like they were going hoarse and then it'd stop for an instant and start again. Back at the same level and pitch.

The husband-to-be had arrived by the time they got Mary Colreavy to her feet. He hammered his way through the cops at the door and put his arms out to her. I don't know did she see him. She just screamed. I never heard screaming like it.

The cops brought me into the street and asked did I want a lift home. I didn't answer them. I just pretended to myself I was a knight of the road in the middle of a journey. And kept thinking if it hadn't been for me going to a party on the night of my brother's funeral none of this would have happened and everyone would have been safe. You couldn't have luck.

Six

Waiting for the Healer

Flying glass gets everywhere. The morning after the shooting a wodge of the stuff was lodged in the fleshy bump between my thumb and index finger. It was the size of a nose stud. The blood had my hand stuck to the sheet when I woke up.

I stayed in bed that day and didn't notice much of what was going on. Heads appeared from time to time. I turned over on my stomach and hugged the pillow. Beetlejuice was in a heap on the floor of the Dandy Diner everywhere I looked. Blood streamed across a carpet to encircle half a banana and dye it dark red. I tried to sleep. Night brought the relief of being able to sit up and look into the dark. And bawl.

In the outside world TV cameras filmed the outside of the Dandy Diner. Clinger and Dalton were still in hospital. A few more people went to Casualty to get cuts looked at. Flying glass.

Mam and Tracey and Liz and Kaya were sitting at the table when I got up the next day. My legs were baby-giraffe wobbly and the light in the kitchen shoved coloured sparks in front of my eyes for a few seconds. Local radio rattled on about the shootings and competed with the noise of the fry. An ad came on for a nightclub where there are no strangers, only friends you have yet to meet.

—Fuck it, I'm going out for the paper. Does anyone want anything from the shop?

I kissed Kaya on the forehead and said I'd be back in ten minutes. I meant it when I said it.

Bernie Sheridan sat on the front wall of the house nearest her and Clinger's caravan. A two times too big parka muffled her up. The fur lining of the hood had been driven three different colours by dampness.

Her ankles had stayed thin. She was struggling to keep her face together and tissues hung down from the stained sleeves of the parka. Bernie pulled out a sheaf of them and feebly blew her nose. She just about managed to produce a thin strand of snot that formed a swaying rope-bridge between her nose and the tissue.

She broke the bridge with another stack of tissues and flung them into the garden behind her. Her nails were bitten down so the stripped skin bled on both little fingers. The skin on her thumb had the look of being left too long in a swimming pool.

—Clinger's all right, Bernie, isn't he?

—Oh, yeah. He'll be out in a couple of days. Yer man got him in the shoulder.

—You seen him?

—I'm going now. Eddie's bringing me. He's awful shook. He was telling me he nearly went back on the drink.

—Tell Clinger I was asking for him.

—Do you want to come? Eddie'll be here in a few minutes. Clinger'd get a fierce kick out of it if you landed down to him.

—No.

Clinger could have been killed. Bernie was wearing his coat. She was living in his caravan. She was carrying his kid. They called him a hero and an example to us all on the local radio. I said no again.

I walked past Hannon's and two other shops. I wanted to be in the town centre.

When I was in National School an old priest landed in from time to time to give us lectures about our lives. He warned us if we didn't watch out we'd turn out to be corner-boys. Corner-boys, he said, leaned against the walls of buildings all day and looked for trouble.

The only men I knew who leaned against walls gathered at the War of Independence monument in Sarsfield Street. They waited there every morning. Alert. Smoking. Never talking to each other. At twenty-five past ten they all disappeared. Sometimes my father and Uncle Jimmy were among them. I asked the oul lad if they were corner-boys. He got a great kick out of it.

—No, no, we're waiting for the healer.

Years later I found out what the healer was. But I still couldn't understand how you could be that desperate for it. Standing there with a view of a dozen pubs. Ready to charge down to the one that opened the door maybe two minutes before the others. I had a feeling one day it would make sense to me. Me and Lydia made sure our front doors were never a second late in swinging open.

The pulling back of a bolt cracked through from McEoin Street and the almost polite creak of an opening door sent twenty men towards Callaghan's on this morning. I followed them. Old Missus Callaghan was still throwing the second half of the door open when we stomped in. Arrival at a safe haven. Smiles all round at the counter. But still no words.

Missus Callaghan's curlers were still in. She padded around behind the bar in a huge pair of Garfield slippers. A little man from St Michael's Heights stood up on the brass rail running under the outside of the bar. The veins in his nose stuck out so clearly it looked like one prick of a needle would do to burst the lot. He put an *Irish Independent* and two cartons of milk on the counter and waved at Missus Callaghan.

—Missus. Missus.

—I'll be with you in a minute, Jody.

—Missus. Missus.

—Oh, all right. He's an awful tyrant, isn't he?

A couple of timid, empathetic chuckles. But no one felt much like laughing. The worst moments are those of the sitting still and waiting. A lob of shouts for shorts and pints of lager to defeat the minutes of suspense which the choice of Guinness would impose. Missus Callaghan gathered some of the previous night's pint glasses from behind the counter. Dregs of stout were left in a few of them. She carefully emptied them into a glass with a lipstick trace on the rim. It came to almost a pint.

—Missus. Missus.

—You'd think when he'd be getting it for nothing he'd be happy.

Missus Callaghan placed the glass under the tap and topped up the concoction with one short blast of porter. Jody accepted it from her with something like grace and gripped both sides of the glass. His hands stretched. Taut. The veins in the back of them forming uneven, knobbly lunar ridges. His fingers like talons. He raised the glass and poured the Guinness down his gullet in less than ten seconds. And carefully licked his lips before walking out the door.

—Thanks, Missus.

—Mind yourself now, Jody.

People seemed more relaxed when he went. I remembered him when he was a Council ganger. Halfway through my second pint a swarthy man with an anchor tattooed on his neck came in. He walked towards the counter. Then he took a few steps back and turned round in a circle a couple of times. The way Kaya did when she tried to make herself dizzy. He sang. Loud.

> Shoe the donkey, shoe the donkey
> We're off to the bog.
> Shoe the donkey, shoe the donkey
> We're off to the bog.

Missus Callaghan was out from behind the counter in a shot.

—Out now. None of that jig-acting.

He was about twice the size of her and he was trembling.

—A drink, Missus Callaghan.

—No drink for you this morning, Ozzie.

—Please can I have a drink, Missus Callaghan?

—No mon, no fun. Where's my *Irish Independent*? Where's the milk?

—I'll go out and get them for you, Missus Callaghan.

—Well, you're too late. At this hour of the morning. Jody has them brought in already. You may go down to Dermot Brennan or Lal McGivney and see has anyone brought them their papers.

The anchor man's face fell in on itself.

—Fuck Jody, fucking cunt, fuck him for a fucking scabby cunt.

—I'll have none of that language in this pub. Get out this minute or I'll get Mr Callaghan down to you.

Her tiny fingers adroitly positioned him to face the door.

He didn't look back as he walked out. Missus Callaghan went down the other end of the bar and talked about cattle prices to an old man in a faded blue suit. Through the glass of the bar door I saw Ozzie pacing up and down the porch. He eased the door open two minutes later and walked back in. Without a song this time.

The people nearest the door didn't even tell him to fuck off when he tried to blodge a few shillings. They just looked straight through him and kept drinking. You could see he didn't fancy coming back into the middle of the pub. But he had to. He landed by my stool.

—Go on, decent man, a poundy woundy, decent man. I knew your father well, decent man.

I trawled the pockets. A pound coin was all I had change-wise. I placed it in his palm. He examined it suspiciously and deposited both hand and coin in the pocket of his jeans. The hems of the jeans were plastered with mud. He thrust out his free hand.

—Decent man. I won't forget you, Ozzie Small doesn't forget his friends, all the shit, you know, I know, fucking OK man, we know.

—Out. Now.

Missus Callaghan was back again. Ozzie Small didn't move at first. A couple of men offered to help her get rid of him. They'd handle him so they would. Guffaws as Ozzie scooted for the door. His hand twitched in his pocket and kept feeling the quid coin. He stopped at the door, threw his head back and howled.

—Shoe the donkey, shoooe the donkey, shooooe the donkey.

The only other time I heard a noise like that was when Lydia and me went to Battersea Dogs' Home to see if we could get a guard-dog for the Horse and Groom. We got a useless grey-muzzled mongrel who enjoyed chasing the joggers in Brockwell Park. Vinnie would let him in at night to sleep in the lounge now I was away.

Ozzie Small won every marksmanship competition in the army when he was in the Plunkett Barracks. He went off to be a mercenary. Every place there was a war Ozzie would be. Angola, Mozambique and Biafra and a rake of other spots. He would send his oul fella a load of cash once in a while. And a letter telling him about all the people he'd killed.

There was a picture behind the bar in Donoghue's. Ozzie sent it to his oul fella one time. It came from an African newspaper. Ozzie being presented with a medal out in the bush by one black fella and other black fellas lying dead at his feet. Biafra. Nigeria. One of the cab drivers who came into the King William was from Nigeria. I was often tempted to ask him if he knew Ozzie Small. But I left it. One of the dead black fellas might have been his brother. You never know where you're talking.

Ozzie was 0800's childhood hero. 0800 was big into this mercenary crack. He used look at the telly news every evening and sulk if there were no wars on. Worried the world would be peaceful by the time he grew up. 0800 used follow Ozzie around when he came home. One day he kept asking him what the Biafrans were like. The Biafrans. The Biafrans. Ozzie turned around and said, with his eyes completely focused on something we couldn't see:

—The Biafrans. I suppose they were like everyone else except you got paid to shoot them.

I killed the rest of the morning in Donoghue's. Joe Donoghue would be in trouble if Pub Spy ever called. Even if the espionage man didn't mind the iron bars on the windows or the barbed wire on the roof he'd surely take exception to the jacks. I wasn't sure if the snails crawling above the piss trough were the same ones that were there before I went to England.

Probably they were relations. But they could be the same ones. Because they were hardy snails. You had to respect them. They inched their way slowly up that damp wall towards the ceiling. And when you took them and put them right at the bottom of the wall again, like I always did, they waited for a second and resumed their journey. And when you came out for your next piss, Brian the Snail would have his way made up the wall again.

Some of the lads would try and piss high up on the wall to send the poor oul snail tumbling into the bottom of the trough. Into the piss. But I didn't think that was fair. It probably killed the snails. Because you never saw one climbing up the silvery wall of the piss trough. Mind you, you never saw one of them stuck in the bottom of it either.

So where did they go?

They spent all their time inching up that wall towards the ceiling. But you never saw one of them hanging down from the ceiling. What was the point? There must be one because they kept going. They were born and lived and died in the jacks of Donoghue's pub in Rathbawn. But they did their best to get on with it. And if you tapped their shell, the little head came out and the extended horns felt around patiently for a few seconds before the snail withdrew back into his house. Politely. Like he was saying:

—Oh, well, nothing drastic, it's a great life if you don't weaken.

Why would anyone want to kill them? I took the snail I'd brought down the wall and placed him back up near the top. I kept my hand on the outside of his shell until I was sure he had a grip on the wall.

Richie Fee's father sat on the stool next to mine. He looked straight in front of himself and made up the price of his next drink in exact coinage when he got below the halfway point of his current one. He drank big cans of cider. With ice in the glass. Every new can brought a request for even more ice in the glass. The glass was three-quarters-way full of jagged cubes. I saluted him as he decanted more cider and shook the glass so it made a noise like a kaleidoscope changing colour.

—It could be worse, Josie.

—Ah, it couldn't, it couldn't, it's terrible.

He popped two tiny blue-and-white capsules into his mouth. Simon McDonagh joined me. He was drinking Lancer. Joe had a store out the back where he kept bottles of booze that were years out of date. He'd pour two of them into a pint glass and take a pound off anyone who didn't mind the smell of their own sick in the morning.

Bakers Lane again. Captain roamed around in front of the fifties and sixties in the Park with his chain chiming against the footpath. There was something a bit pathetic about him now. He looked disorientated. He couldn't work out why Beetlejuice hadn't turned up the last couple of days. You could see that.

The National Schools had just got off for the day. The Park was full of parents walking tiny kids back to small houses. Same as it ever was. Same as it had been when my most valuable possession had been my Spider Man flask.

Except it was the men who walked the kids home now. The mammies went home once with the kids and waited the couple of hours for the daddies to come home from the Council gang or the ambulance factory.

Now men stopped on the cracked footpaths and passed on the gossip. They'd sit in front of the telly and wait the couple of hours for wives and girlfriends to finish contract-cleaning jobs, work in Rathbawn Textiles or a stint in the Dutch factory that made luxury cigars for the export market and only employed women.

Liz and Francie and Mam drank tea in the kitchen. They told me Kaya was having a nap and went straight back to their conversation. I went into the sitting-room. The blues and reds of the television seemed like an intrusion, so I rooted around to see if there was anything to read. Anything with words in it. Words I could put between my thoughts and my life.

Don't think of Lydia whatever you do, Paul.

My chin was all covered with dribble when I woke up on the couch. The clock told me the day wasn't next nor near nearly over. I had to brush my teeth before I went into the kitchen but even the Sloosh didn't remove the flavour of irregularity from my mouth.

—Snap.

A look of intense concentration in Kaya's face. Mam blinked when I walked in but neither of them looked up.

—Snap.

Kaya had a big pile of cards in front of her. Mam had enough for a poker hand. I pulled a chair over to the table. I felt I should say something.

—Snap.

Mam smiled at me. The smile was in her eyes as well. I know because I checked.

—I'm winning, Dad.

—Good.

I didn't say anything else. I just hoped Kaya would win this game soon so I could play in the next one. Mam had taken Kaya's hair out of the corn-row and tied it up in a pony-tail.

—Snap.

A six and a nine had fallen on to the table in quick succession. Kaya told me Granny Kelly wasn't very good at cards when Mam went to wet the tea.

—We're having a nice day.

I nodded. I could hear the hot-water cylinder bubbling away in the background.

—Kaya said she'd like a bath.

Kaya was eeking as Mam poured a jug of warm water on

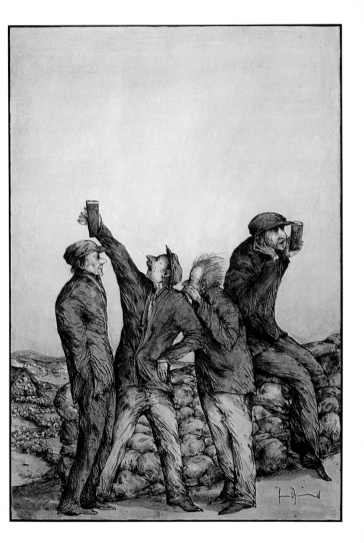

Gertrude Degenhardt

Was born in New York, and grew up in Berlin
She lives and works
On the Irish West Coast and in the Rhine Valley

»Paradise Lost«

Overleaf is shown a reproduction
Of the colour aquatint etching
»Paradise Lost«
Which has appeared in a limited edition of 200 copies
On 350 gramme mould-made paper
The size of the four copper plates is 500 x 350 mm
The format of the paper is 720 x 530 mm
Each etching is numbered and signed by the artist

The drypoint sequence of the cycle
»Vagabondage Ad Mortem«
Will be displayed in its entirety

You are invited to the opening of the exhibition

»Paradise Lost«

Imagines by

Gertrude Degenhardt

At The Kenny Gallery, Middle Street, Galway
On Thursday, September 12th at 6 for 6.30 p.m.
The exhibition will be opened by

Tom Kenny

Shown will be brush drawings, gouaches, and
Etchings of the cycle

»Paradise Lost«

The exhibition will be from September 12th to
November 1st 1996

Opening hours
Monday to Saturday 9 a.m. to 6 p.m.

The Kenny Gallery

Middle Street, Galway, Ireland,
Phone (0 91) 56 10 21, Fax (0 91) 56 85 44

Gertrude Degenhardt

»Vagabondage Ad Mortem«
Musicians of Death

The cycle is accompanied by a
Multilingual catalogue book
Comprising full-page reproductions of
Gouaches, brush drawings, drypoints, and lithographs

Format 160 x 230 mm, thread-stitched and
Bound in cloth, 140 pages, limited to
1000 copies

The special edition is limited to
100 copies, each copy in slip case
Together with a drypoint etching

Edition GD, Klosterstraße 1 A, D-55124 Mainz
Phone (0 61 31) 4 25 23, Fax (0 61 31) 4 57 17

her head when I walked into the bathroom. A Johnson's Baby Shampoo slick polluted the water. A battered yellow plastic duck valiantly surfed the waves until a delighted splash of Kaya's right hand sent it tumbling on to its side.

Jesus, the little sizeen of her. In the bath with her eyes shut dead tight, like I told her to do, so not a drop of shampoo would creep under the lids.

—It'll make you cry if it gets in your eyes.

—I don't want to cry.

Her fearfully flickering eyes. The pinkness of her tiny steam-surrounded body. These things made me want to speak to her. To reassure her. To tell her there was a theory of everything and it said the job was Oxo with the world. Kaya had a tiny bump at the bottom of her backbone. I always felt I should have been able to smooth it out.

—You all right, love?

—Yeah . . . Dad?

—Yeah.

—Ask Granny if there's any bubbles.

Mam needed two goes to open the cabinet over the sink. It crawled with razors, aftershave and mouthwash. Johnny's things. She footered around for a bit before she triumphantly dislodged a long, blue plastic bottle. A couple of Wilkinson Sword razor blades toppled into the sink.

—If it's bubbles she wants, it's bubbles she'll get.

—Ta, Gran.

Kaya smiled. With those impossibly perfect small teeth I'd have to creep in and dislodge from under her pillow in a couple of years. They would be small and white with a little trail of dried blood. The baby teeth she'd never have again.

The liquid did its best to foment some bubbles in the still water. Kaya felt around with her hands and squealed with delight as she made contact with the first clump of foam. She liked bubbles. Got months out of a simple yoke for blowing soap rings. Slobbered Aero on a pair of new white trousers the day after Kerrie bought them for her. Mam thrust the long, blue plastic bottle happily into my hand.

—Do you remember this?

The grinning face with the two happy dimples on the cheeks. The kerchief around the neck. Like a faithful old friend. Matey. I thought they'd stopped making it. Nah. To tell the truth, I hadn't thought about Matey Bubble Bath at all for quite a while.

Dead Johnny and me used get a bottle of it each at Christmas. Big highlight. No cod. Two major fucking bubble freaks. Saturday-night baths. After *Jim'll Fix It*. So many bubbles in the bath you couldn't see the water. The pair of us in that small white bath I wouldn't be able to stretch out fully in now. But me and the dead man once fitted perfectly in it. Both of us. Hard to imagine that. Like resting both your elbows on top of a wall you once couldn't imagine seeing over.

Johnny and me in the bath. A clear picture. In colour to make up for it only being in my mind. Me down the end away from the taps. Privilege of the elder to be spared the hassle of trying to lean back without making contact with either the shiver of the cold or the scorch of the hot.

Me and Johnny. Two little boys. With our two little toys dangling into the water. Whatever there was to dangle at that age. The only man I'd ever been naked in a bath with. And I thought nothing of it. At an age when you'd live in fear of someone seeing the colour of your jocks. That had to count. Else nothing stood for anything.

There were too many baths and shared shinguards with the Manchester United logo on them to let this lie. Mam used wrap towels around our heads, swathing them round in circles and letting the ends trail down our backs.

—Make me into an Arab, Mam, make me into an Arab.

I needed to get out of the house and back into the present. I wondered if whoever had knocked off Johnny and Beetlejuice would come for me. There was no reason they should. But I was still scared. There was no reason they shouldn't. I walked for a good fifteen minutes before I realized I was hitting towards the Diamond.

The Rob Alls drank in the Westerner. The barrels neatly stacked against the front wall had a habit of going through the front window on major public holidays and important family occasions. I wanted to go in there and tell someone I'd known Beetlejuice. But my determination was ebbing even before I saw the row outside.

—There's no rapists on our side of the family.

—You got no satisfaction your last time in court.

—You're a whore for every man on the Diamond.

—And you don't know whether it's a child you're carrying or a coffin.

The last comment was pitched at a tall woman who was several months pregnant and had lazy, deep-brown eyes. The two sides shuffled closer to each other. The woman who'd done most of the slagging caught hold of the pregnant woman's hair and screeched:

—It'll be fucking born with TB.

A man jumped out from behind her and into the middle of the crowd. He tried two of those windmilling push-off-with-one-foot-and-lash-into-the-air-with-the-other high kicks Bruce Lee used do and fell on his arse after the second one. Another man threw off his shirt. A red-raw scar ran down his back like a giant question mark. He pulled the other man up off the ground and punched him. The pregnant woman tried to get to the Westerner's door. She was shielded by a man who'd pulled a butcher's knife out of his coat and was jabbing it in front of him.

I walked past the edge of the beating match. I didn't pass much heed. They were all cousins. They'd make it up after a bit. A squad would arrive, have a look and drive away again.

A heavy man with wisps of hair clinging to a red scalp sat on the footpath a few yards up from the Westerner with a six-pack of Heineken balanced in his lap. Another six-pack sprawled in the gutter alongside a rake of shards of glass.

He emptied another bottle into him and smashed it against the ground. Tears streamed down his face. I knew he was one of Beetlejuice's brothers. I couldn't think of his name. He looked like a man in hell. A wasp hovered around his mouth. He puffed a breath outwards and watched intently as it continued its mesmerized dance in front of his face. I turned back for home at the outside edge of the Diamond and walked back by the Canal Line. I wished I'd gone to Noelie Reilly's removal. But I knew I wouldn't go to his funeral the next day. The Rob Alls had their space like we had ours.

Myself and Mam ended up watching a late-night horror where the vampire was far less frightening than the checked suits worn by the hero. A horn sounded outside. We kept our eyes on the screen. The horn sounded again.

—Take a look out the window, Paul. That sounds like it's outside our gate.

It went for the third time as I peeled back the corner of the curtains and looked out.

—Save it for the fucking wife, I said to try and get a laugh from Mam.

Also to hide the fact that my heart was gone up to high doh. She must have heard the tremor in my voice.

—Is it for here?

The car was outside our gate. One hazard-warning light flickered. One man sat in the car. A circle of orange light moved towards the driver's seat as he brought the cigarette lighter to his mouth. The tip of the fag glowed. I knew he knew we were looking at him. And so on. There was another flash of light when he opened his door.

—I'll call the guards, Paul.

—Don't be daft, Mam.

I recognized him. Beetlejuice's brother. The one who had been breaking green bottles on the footpath. He stopped at our gate.

—Where's Paul Kelly? I want to speak to Paul Kelly. Come out, Paul, I want to have a chat to you.

His voice was silted with the thickness around the edges drinking brings. The lager clung around the shape of the words like a crust. But he spoke deliberately. The way a cat picks its steps. Mam joined me at the window.

—That's Bumper Reilly. There's a knife down in the bottom of the wardrobe in your room if you want it. Don't go out to him, that fella isn't all in it.

—Paul, come out to me, will you?

He wasn't coming any further than the gate. Something in his voice connected with the tears tumbling down his face outside the Westerner. I opened the front door and walked out. The night was silent except for the sound of a cat either fighting or having it away. The noise made me jump. I hadn't the knife with me because I knew if a situation came up where it was needed it wouldn't be any use to me.

—Come out to the car.

Bumper offered me a cigarette and pulled the lighter out from the dashboard again. I took it from him and lit the fag myself in case his hands slipped and jabbed the lighter into my eye. *The Leuuve Zone* was on the car radio. Bumper knocked it off. He leaned against the steering wheel and didn't look at me when he spoke.

—I didn't come in 'cause I thought your mother has enough trouble to deal with at the moment.

—She wouldn't have minded.

—All the same.

He blew two expert smoke rings and started the engine. 'Love' was tattooed on the fingers of his right hand. He hadn't got around to having 'Hate' done on his left.

—Sorry about your brother.

—Thanks. I'm sorry about yours. Noelie always said Johnny was a sound oul sketch. So what are we going to do about it?

—. . .

—Come on. Tell me.

—You tell me.

—Fuck you.

He tipped his cigarette. Tiny sparks cut through the dark.

—What can we do?

The butt fell on the floor. An acrid smell of old tobacco lived in the car. Bumper leaned back in his seat and folded his arms. He unfolded them, and jabbed a finger into my chest. Hard. I winced but didn't flinch and hoped the dark hid my facial expression. He jabbed a second time. I moved my shoulder round so I wasn't facing him straight on any more.

—Someone killed your brother. And then they shot my brother like an oul bad dog because he was your brother's friend. Fuck it, we can't have it said that we let someone get away with that.

— . . .

—Are you a man or a mouse? There's hoors someplace knows who killed Noel and John. Whoever it is, I'm getting them. Your brother was killed and all, are you on for it?

—I don't know.

—Your brother, like. I know the Kellys is no daws. I want you to help me on this. The rest of our crowd wouldn't do it right. But you and me could. Are you in or not? Shit or get off the pot.

—How are we going finding out who did it?

—We'll find out. Word'll be got. Come on, we'll have an oul couple of scoops and we'll work it out.

—It's half two. Where will you get pints at this hour?

Bumper gunned the car through the Park. Half a dozen

youngsters in debs' dresses and tuxedoes wandered bemusedly up Main Street towards the taxi rank. The night was quiet apart from them. Their primary colours shone in the rear-view mirror as we drove out to the Diamond.

A few murmurs and a lot of movement when Bumper battered the side-door of the Westerner. A chair was dragged across the floor and someone stepped up on top of it. A dimly lit face peered down at us from the small rectangle of glass above the door.

—It's very late, Bumper.

—Is it fuck late. You have a gang inside. Let us in, for fuck's sake, Sean.

The place was pitch-black. We might as well have been down a hole.

—Fuck's sake, Sean, son, if I fall here you'll be paying compo.

—You can't pay out what you haven't got. We had the light of the telly but you hammering the door finished that.

Sean fumbled in his pocket for the remote.

—If I leave it out of me sight, someone whips it. Ye'll all be sorry when there's no more telly.

On came the telly. The sudden light revealed a smiling Bumper with a smaller remote at the end of his outstretched arm.

—Abracadabra.

A couple of men appeared from behind the counter. A few more walked out of the ladies' jacks.

—The show must go on.

—Whose pint is whose?

—Put the video back on.

—Mine is the full one there.

The stools were arranged in a semi-circle in front of the television. Twenty men sitting in the dark all looking at a woman young enough to be a granddaughter to some of them. And her dressed in a French maid's outfit and getting belaboured by men, women and the odd inanimate implement. The manky green paint on the wall behind her was enough to put me off. A microphone on the end of a stick periodically bobbed into view at the top of the screen.

Bumper got bored with the action. He tapped me on the shoulder and nodded towards a corner of the pub. We sat in the semi-dark with only the occasional shout from the video viewers to distract us.

—He might be a honky but he's hung like a donkey.

—Now you're sucking diesel.

—Go on, use the vibrator.

The light of his cigarette lit up Bumper's eyes. They were what I could see best.

—Are you game anyways? Will you team up with me . . . for Johnny's sake?

—I suppose so. I'll make no promises.

—You're a sound man. You're cleverer than me too. I'd say you're a bit of a brain-box at the back of it all.

—I'm not too clever in fairness, Bumper.

—Stop the lights, will you? You're able to mind yourself. I'd know by you. We're a team. We won't stop till we've sorted every last fuckbag out. A team, son, like Starsky and Hutch.

Starsky. Johnny's tongue and teeth used clash on awkward words sometimes. If he'd been made say it a hundred times it would still have come out the same way.

—Skarsky.

Skarsky. Quesgyans. I knew I could tell Bumper to fuck off. I knew I could get out of this and go back to England and the life I had. Except I didn't have a lot of the life I had any more. The decision was made even though I knew it was a wrong one. Because I wasn't sure. And Bumper seemed to be sure of what he was going doing. Of what we were going doing.

It's all about revenge. About not letting it be said someone got the better of you. The thought had jumped through the phone line the second Uncle Jimmy told me Johnny was dead. It had followed me in taxis, a boat and trains and walked beside me in the Park. It was a flicker but all that was missing was something to set it alight. Or make it explode.

I needed Bumper.

Bumper was still thinking about revenge when everyone else had left the pub. Sean took away our glasses. Ten minutes later he came down and swabbed our table with a wet cloth that made it dirtier. Ten more minutes passed.

—Come on, lads. Time to hit the road. It's not a hotel I'm running here.

Bumper walked up to the counter.

—Another couple of drinks and we'll go then. Come on, Sean, and get one for yourself.

—Bumper, good man, will you go home? I'm falling down with tiredness.

—Go on, Sean, have an oul drink.

—Sure, ye've had all evening to drink. Save your money, I'll be open first thing in the morning.

—Can we have a short, Sean.

There was no question mark there. Sean turned his back.

—No. Go home.

—After all our family spend here, spent here this evening. You're only a fucking arsehole, Sean. That's all you are, Sean. A fucking arsehole and a bollocks.

Sean turned around again and gripped the counter with both hands while trying to pretend he was smiling.

—After what happened in here this evening, I owe nothing to your family. After what was tried to be done to me.

—My brother is dead. Noelie is fucking dead, Sean. And you refuse me a drink when I need a drink and my brother dead above in the house. My brother, Sean, that's some fucking respect to my family.

Bumper took a hatchet out of his jacket. He swung short-armed with it and clipped Sean on the elbow.

—Fuck you, Sean.

—Me fucking arm, get out to fuck or I'm calling the cops.

—Fuck's sake, Bumper, stop it, man.

—You'll call no fucking cops.

The hatchet swung in a powerful downward arc. There was an emphatic crunch and a splitting of timber as it embedded itself in the counter. Bumper rubbed his right hand as we undid the bolts of the side-door. Sean was still hopping around in pain behind the counter. His impassioned 'Fucks' rang out over the Diamond since we never bothered to close the door after us.

The debutantes were still waiting at the taxi rank. They hugged each other to keep warm. All the boys were down to their shirts now. Tuxedoes hung over their companions' fake-tanned shoulders.

I realized I was panicking just before I got into bed. Kaya. I had a feeling something might have happened to her and I was worried enough to push her bedroom door straight in instead of nudging it ajar.

She was sleeping like a log. Huddled up in the bed Tracey and Liz once shared. Breathing calmly through her nostrils. Her thumb in her mouth. That's bad for the teeth, isn't it? I coaxed it out of her mouth. She stirred slightly.

A tiny trail of spittle was on my index finger where I had removed Kaya's thumb from her baby teeth. The feel of that dampness was my last sensation before I panned out.

I dreamed it again.

I am young and I am walking along this country road wearing a stripy T-shirt and a pair of shorts. It is a dry, dusty road surrounded by fields of green grass. There's a heat haze coming up off the road and I feel my tongue swelling up and hurting me because it is so dry.

I come across a pump. One of those old blue parish

pumps. I pull the handle and water flows out of it. The water is silver like brand-new ten-pence coins and sparkling in the sun like on ads and it is the most refreshing drink I've ever had.

Every moment of the dream is with me when I wake up. But what annoys me is not knowing where it comes from. They had those pumps out the country one time. But I never saw one in Rathbawn. And I never drank from one.

Seven

A Fool to Yourself

The Rs vibrated on Mam's tongue like the rattle of building labourers' teeth outside Camden Town Tube on a frosty winter morning.

—What did he want, Paul? I was terrified.

Her 'terrified' sounded like the exact meaning of the word.

—Nothing. He just needed to have a pint and talk about Johnny and Beetlejuice.

—What about them?

—Nothing, really. He just wanted an oul chat about funeral arrangements and things.

—Paul, I hope you're not getting involved with that fella in anything.

I shook my head as though this was the most ludicrous suggestion in the world. Which it was although it was true.

—Ah, Mam, he's a married man.

—You know well what I mean.

Outside the window it was Saturday. That meant a lot less in the Park than it had one time. Mam wouldn't let go.

—Are you listening to me, Paul?

—I am, of course, but I don't know why you're talking at me.

—Don't get in with that fella, that's all I'm telling you. He's cracked. You know what happened with him and Simon McDonagh.

—No.

—Simon's young lad Barney bet one of Bumper's kids for making faces at him.

—What age is Barney?

—Barney McDonagh is sixteen. Bumper's young boy is seven but he's a bould stump all the same. Bumper went down to McDonagh's and told Simon to send Barney out so he could batter him. Simon wouldn't so Bumper pasted him on his own doorstep.

—Simon is no angel.

—Simon sent Bumper a solicitor's letter and Bumper posted it back to him with two lumps of crap in the envelope. He saw Mary Ann McDonagh in the shopping centre and he says to her, 'Isn't it fierce what the lawyers are writing these days, it's pure shite.'

I tried to take a logical viewpoint. Bumper's. It was his son after all. What could he do?

—Bumper got hold of young Barney in O'Connell Crescent on Bonfire Night. He put a wire snare around his neck and destroyed him. Barney went to England.

I wondered if the hatchet was still sticking up at that peculiar angle from the Westerner's counter. It was twelve o'clock. I felt not too bad. I'd been sleeping better than I had for years. My body moulded naturally into my old bed. Could be that said something about where home was. Could be it didn't.

—Mam, where's Kaya?

—Oh, aye, I should have said that to you. I meant to say it to you first thing you got up but I was all worried about this Bumper Reilly caper.

—There's nothing wrong with her, Mam, is there?

—No, no. It's just Tracey was going into town shopping and she asked Kaya if she wanted to come in with them and Kaya said yes. I wanted to wake you up but Tracey said to leave you asleep.

—She would.

I tried to sound annoyed but the only annoyance I felt was at my lack of annoyance. Kaya would be all right. She would understand in the end. I had a mission to carry out. Me and Bumper Reilly. I needed him to get my own back. So I didn't want to hear about wire snares and shite in envelopes.

Isn't it what being an Irishman or any man is all about? Standing up for your rights. Not letting it be said that people got the better of you. Kaya would understand. In the end.

Joe Donoghue himself was behind the bar in Donoghue's. He came down to talk to me. *Football Focus* was on so we communicated in oohs, aahs and winces at the goals, saves and sendings off of the European round-up. We looked at each other the second *Football Focus* ended.

—You did well in the oul pub game beyond, Paul.

—Did all right. Where would I leave it? Wasn't I studying you all these years?

—You're like your oul fella, full of shite. I'd say those good English pubs wouldn't be like this one.

—A lot of them were more like the Westerner.

Joe chuckled and rolled Old Holborn lovingly into fag paper. It made a fat cigarette he lodged between yellow fingers. I held a match out for him.

—I'd say there was wild sport in the Westerner last night.

—I'd say there was all right, Joe.

—Comanche country, that place. D'you know the Reillys

shot the crow in every pub in town last night before they hit there?

—Including here?

—They paid here but there was nearly a fucking riot over what happened in the Westerner. They landed oul bollocks Sean with four hundred in forged twenties.

Bumper walked in five minutes later. Joe looked at me and then looked disappointed when Bumper shouted two pints and asked me how the head was after last night. Joe made a production out of holding Bumper's ten note up to the light.

—I made it meself this morning, Joe.

Bumper clinked his pint glass against mine.

—Joe was taking no chance with that tenner.

—Ah, well, there's a lot of forgeries around these days.

—I know. I bought those twenties for six pound each in Dublin. I thought Sean would be too stupid to notice them. Come on. We have business to take care of.

—I have to be home for the afternoon. To see the daughter.

—You're in or you're out. Act the white man.

I hoped we wouldn't meet Tracey or Kaya in the street. Tracey wouldn't be impressed. Or scared. She was a walking bitch sometimes. It wouldn't be the worst thing for Kaya to turn out like her.

I saw the grey-faced man with the matching suit locking the door of his Mazda 323 the second we walked into the Market Yard. I knew his phizog from the *Champion*. He knew Bumper's face from somewhere too. He already had the car locked. But now he gazed deep into the door and kept twisting the key in the lock. Unlocking. Locking. Unlocking. Locking. Unlocking. Locking. And looking over at Bumper out the side of his eye. Bumper winked at me.

—Have a dekko at this. Come on, we'll walk past the fucker.

The man in the suit looked straight down. At the key. At the lock. At his feet. Down into the ground and into the town sewerage system.

—Grrrrrr.

The growling came from deep in Bumper's throat. Maybe even up from his stomach. The man's fingers were white around the keys. He didn't look up even though Bumper was just a couple of feet away from his ear. Bumper coughed carefully to clear his throat and growled again.

—Grrrrrr.

He clapped me on the back when he'd done it a couple more times. His voice was cheerful.

—Come on over to the car. See you around, Mr Byrne.

I knew the face but the name or who he was still wouldn't come to me.

—Mr Byrne. The Housing Officer with the Council.

—So. What's the crack?

Bumper got an angry horn blast from a driver who reckoned it was his right of way. We slowed down and Bumper rolled down the window.

—What the fuck are you at, son? Don't hoot your fucking horn at me. I'm Bumper Reilly, who are you? Who the fuck knows who you are?

We were outside the town before Bumper's temper was down enough for him to tell me about the Housing Officer.

—I fell behind with the oul rent. Well, I didn't pay it for six years. Money wasn't great and it's sort of the first thing you put off paying. So Mr Byrne wrote me a letter and said they had a court order to get me kicked out of the house.

—You hardly went.

—I phoned him and told him I'd kill anyone who came near the house and that I knew where he lived and I'd burn his house down with him in it. So he said he'd do a deal. If I paid the rent from now on, and added on forty quid a week, I could stay in the house.

—Jesus, forty quid is serious dosh.

—It is when you think about it. So whenever I saw Mr Byrne in town, I'd go over and growl at him, 'Grrrrrr, Grrrrrr, Grrrrrr.' I kept it going for a while and then I got a letter asking me to come into the Council and meet him and not say anything about it. I got to sit in one of those groovy swivel chairs in his office. I was picturing the shape the chair would make when I put it through the window with Mr Byrne still sitting on it. I was sure he was going saying he had the pigs set on me.

—He's scared of his fucking shite of you.

—He is that. He told me if I stopped growling at him the whole time he'd pull the extra money down to ten plus the rent. Grand, I said. But I still growl at him the odd time just so he remembers to keep the right side of me.

—Are you paying the rent since?

—Of course I am. All I needed was an oul reminder.

—Where are we going?

—On a bit of a trek around the county. I do it the odd time. You see a bit of the world that way. Drinking in the same town the whole time reminds me of being in jail.

Bumper parked the car on the main street and only street of Sheepwalk. A village with one shop, a sub-post office and three pubs. We walked past the first two pubs and towards the third, which stood beside an ancient grey church. A weather-beaten statue of a surprisingly sexy-looking Virgin Mary lurked in front of the church. Bumper rabbited on with the stumbling delight of someone who doesn't get to practise their talking too often.

—What I done with Mr Byrne was I cowed him. That's my theory of life. You have to cow people. You have to spend all your time cowing people or you're bet. You end up cowed yourself.

'The Sheepwalk Inn' hung across the front of the pub in thick, green plastic lettering.

—Do they walk out again, Bumper?

—Only the unattractive ones.

Two old men sat at opposite ends of the counter. They cradled glasses of spirits and looked resignedly at a football match on the big colour television over the bar.

—God bless all here.

Bumper was defying someone to tell him to fuck off. But that person wasn't here. The two old-stagers just looked at the glasses. They seemed to be pondering the significance of the thumbprint patterns on the outside. It was five minutes before the landlady brushed her way past the strips of bright plastic that screened the kitchen from the bar. The same sort of strips hung down at the doors of Pearce and Prunty Bookmaker's and Soho sex shops.

—How are they all in Sheepwalk this weather, Missus Shannon?

Bumper was teasing and he knew the answer he was going to get. But he kept trying to knock some chat out of the landlady. She cut him dead every time. He whispered to me when she made another sortie into the kitchen to prepare unrequested toasted sandwiches for the grumpy old men.

—You see can you get chatting to her? There's something I want to ask her about.

My luck was no better. Cut. She decided to talk when we came near the end of our drinks.

—Are ye from the town, boys? My son P.J. was living in the town up to last week but he's gone out of it now. He's at home for the moment. He got sick and he had to give up his job.

—That's a terror. The way things is gone these days, you can hardly afford to give up any job. But, sure, nothing is worth damaging your health over.

Bumper sounded like he might even know what he was on about.

We were there a while. Every time Bumper heard feet

touch the gravel outside he flicked a glance at the door. It turned from a glance to a gaze when the drunk man walked in. More a swagger than a walk. The man's light-blue T-shirt didn't make much effort to contain the muscles on his chest and upper arms. He would have been an impressive sort of a cut of a skin if it hadn't been for the sickly yellow-white belly peeping from underneath the T-shirt and the look spreading outwards from his eyes The look of a hunted man. The voice of one too.

—Any cunt looking for me, any fucking hoor of a bastarding bollocks looking for me in this shithole, Mammy?

The last word had so much scorn towed behind, it sounded like the name of the Turkish buck who stuck one on the Pope. One of the old geezers clicked his tongue against the roof of his mouth. The other sucked his teeth.

—Don't use that sort of language in my pub, P.J.

It took about a second for Bumper to set his pint on the counter, leap off his stool and put P.J. in a shoulder-lock. P.J. tried to bolt but he hadn't a hope. Bumper stuck a whisper in his ear. A razor-blade earring hung from the lobe. P.J. pointed to the jacks door. Bumper held it open for P.J. and bowed. A smell of seventy-two years' piss wafted into the bar. Missus Shannon's face twitched a couple of times under her make-up.

—He's not a guard, is he, your friend?

—He's some looking cop in fairness.

The signs on the telegraph poles said there was a Wedding Fayre on. In the blue-and-white hotel in the middle of Newtownmanor. The Black and Tans once burned down the town creamery and then had seven shades of shit shot out of them a couple of miles down the road. Someone who'd once been famous on RTE was droning on in the ballroom about going-away outfits. Nervous women in peach, white and pink outfits that made them look like walking layered meringues were smoking in the foyer and practising their promenading at the same time.

—Paul, go into the bar and wait for me. I'll only be a couple of minutes. I have to see a man about a dog.

Posters all around the bar previewed coming attractions.

BERNIE KILBRIDE AND THE DEPORTEES.

Bernie Kilbride looked soulfully into the distance. The small green Aer Lingus jumbo in the photo seemed to be coming out of his ear.

Bumper put his head in the door of the bar after a bit.

—Chop, chop.

I pointed to my pint glass. It was half full. No, we're not getting into that again.

—Bring it with you.

I did. Bumper was shaking hands with a man in a chef's uniform when I got into the hall. Your man even had that long white hat that looks like an elongated pastry case. Or a telescope. Dark blood dripped from the man's nose. It stained his uniform. He would definitely need a biological powder. But he tried to smile. Bumper shook his hand.

We bought American fried chicken, Mexican onion rings and French fries before we left Newtownmanor. Bumper went a roundabout way into Cordrum so we had all eaten well before we got there. It would only have been ten miles by the main road. We came out a side road and there we were. Opposite the county dump. The caravans on the halting site nestled in the shade of the piles of rubbish which seemed to spring naturally from the earth to form great Gothic cathedrals of degradation.

—Out of the way, Missus Knacker.

Bumper spoke through his teeth as a woman ran out of a caravan and snatched a naked child in off the road. We parked opposite a shop that sold Bibles and old-style briar pipes.

—We'll walk from now on. It'll be handier. There's nothing only fucking traffic in this town.

A big sheet of paper behind the bar in O'Hanlon's asked us to buy lines to support the Prisoners' Dependent Fund so we did. The pub was freezing cold. It was built to hold five hundred people. But it never had. A Yank built it because he was a millionaire. When it finally opened he wasn't one any more. Bumper talked to a few men who were organizing a bus to a Cordrum Town cup match in Dublin. A band set up their gear and looked around unenthusiastically at the wide open spaces they were going to be facing even if ten times more people turned up. He asked the location of a couple of heads. No joy. We left when the band started tuning up.

—They'd tell you fucking nothing.

Bumper kicked the front wall of O'Hanlon's. Little tufts of grey dust puffed up and adhered to the toe of his shoe.

—They wouldn't give you the steam of their piss.

The other time I was in O'Hanlon's my oul fella and Uncle Jimmy bought me Cidona and introduced me to men and women with strange accents that sounded like a dog barking. The men and women told me I'd grow up to be a fine-looking Irishman. I remember the chairs gliding through the air after the winning raffle ticket was drawn.

—And the winning ticket is an orange ticket, number . . .

—Boo! Boo!

They shouted the actual word *Boo*!

—Orange bastards. Orange bastards.

—Draw it again. Orange bastards.

—I'm getting me fucken prize. Get out of me fucken way.

—Orange bastards. Draw it again.

—Out of me fucken way.

—Stand your ground like an Irishman.

The barman from O'Hanlon's shouted down the street after us:

138

—Lads, lads, hang on, Bumper, we were only taking the piss. Don't be such a sore frigger.

Bumper breathed out through his nose. The barman walked towards us. He still had a red-and-white-checked dishcloth in his hand.

—Go out to the Canal Bar. The crew that knows about them things is out there.

It was a mile out to the Canal Bar. We decided to walk so we'd be in some form for action when we got out there. The drink was catching up on us.

Everyone usually clocks you the sec you walk into pubs like the Canal Bar. But no one noticed us because a middle-aged woman was doing a 'Take Your Pick' on the stage when we arrived. She was offered sixty pounds for the envelope in her hand. The collective scream of the pub told her to keep going. She bottled the game and settled for sixty. The compère opened the envelope. A cheque for five hundred quid was in it. The woman looked dazed. The compère had to call her back to give her the sixty. He pressed the notes against her hand. The knowledge of what the five hundred could have done in her life seemed to take the power out of her fingers. She shook her head and bundled the dosh into her handbag.

—You sit at the bar and watch my back.

Bumper walked across the dance-floor. He passed between two grey-haired jiving women, detached one and waltzed a couple of steps gracefully with her before spinning her back to her mate. The woman smiled. Four black-haired women who looked like sisters sat at a short-strewn table on the edge of the dance-floor. Two men who were chatting them fucked off when Bumper approached. He asked the bar-boy to bring them down a round. A couple of the women lit cigarettes.

I got beckoned over after a couple of minutes. Bumper did a Pope sign with his right hand and the woman he'd been talking to sat up and reached her hand across the table to me.

—Paul, this is Sylvia. Sylvia, this is Paul.

Bumper deliberately talked about the weather and shut Sylvia up any time she tried to ask me a question. Sylvia's son landed over. He had a plastic football under his arm and threw it to Bumper, whose header sent the ball hopping across the dance-floor. The gossan ducked past the forest of jiving legs and neatly chipped the ball up into his hand. Not a bad effort at all for a squirt who was hardly five. His mother won a bottle of whiskey in the raffle. Her son kicked the ball against the speakers at the side of the stage.

Bumper was full of silence on the way back into town.

—That Jason lad is a good youngster, Bumper.

—He's Noelie's son.

I didn't say anything else for a while. Bumper lit a fag in front of a men's-wear shop on Centenary Square. Lying down on the footpath and sleeping there seemed a good idea. It seemed the logical thing. I looked in the window of the shop and tried to think of reasons to keep walking. Not the easiest thing to do.

—They have nice oul gear in this place, Bumper.

—Do they?

He came level with me and looked in the window at both the clothes and his own reflection. He rolled his shoulders a couple of times.

—That leather jacket is classy.

Bumper nodded agreement and shoved me backwards suddenly. I tried to put up a guard and thought about making a run for it. He turned around. *Smasssssssh*. Bumper was in the shop window, picking little bits of glass off his clothes. He whipped the jacket off an awkward-looking dummy. The dummy looked cold in his short-sleeved shirt.

—How do I look? Does it suit me?

—Come on to fuck. There's people over the other side of the street, come on to fuck, for fuck's sake.

What had been left of the shop window got kicked out on to the footpath before Bumper jumped down and set off at as much of a sprint as we could manage. He held his right arm up to his nose and sniffed exaggeratedly.

—You know, Paul, you can't beat the smell of a new leather jacket. *Go raibh mile maith agat*, Mr Paki.

I had a stitch in my side but it was Bumper who stopped. He leaned against another shop window and put his hands up to his face. Murphy's Butchers. If you went by the pictures on the plastic sign over the door they provided prime lamb and Alsatian.

—Pleased to meet you, meat to please you.

Still, Bumper was hardly going to decide he fancied two pounds of sausages at this hour. He was hardly going to. We didn't have any place to cook them. Unless he wanted them for when he went home. He shook with laughter and kept wiping his eyes with a grubby green handkerchief embossed with someone else's initials.

—Jesus, boss, if you saw your face. Fuck's sake, boss, fuck's sake.

I started laughing myself. I had to. The set of himself in that expensive leather jacket and the price tag still hanging off it. And the big size of him laughing and laughing again. Both of us laughing. Giggling. Chuckling. Chortling. Guffawing.

—I'm a mad cunt, you know, Paul. You know that, don't you? You never know what I'm going to do. You don't have a clue. You're there thinking to yourself, what is the mad cunt going to do next, and you don't have a clue.

I saw the headlights had been left on before Bumper did. The battery was flatter than Norfolk.

—Right, Mr Fucking Mad, what are we going to do now?

—Steal another one. I didn't have that one insured so it's hardly much loss to me.

We picked a corner of the shopping centre carpark where the overhead lights had been broken. I often wonder what sort of *ludramaun* leaves their cars in one of those backlots late at night anyways. How and ever.

—What about this BMW, Bumper? It's a grand-looking yoke.

—I'm looking for an Opel. I want an Opel.

—Why?

—Because Opels is the easiest car to steal. It's easy knowing you never robbed a car.

The way he said it made me feel ashamed. As if I couldn't read or write and someone had found me out. He smashed a front window, hot-wired the car in a few seconds and asked me to drive because he was too drunk to.

I sat in and revved up the engine. Bumper jumped into the back. He didn't trust himself to get all the glass off the passenger seat. I hoped he wouldn't fall asleep. I wouldn't feel safe if he did. He leaned out over the seat and rooted in the glove compartment. Nothing there only a brown lipstick, a scissors and a pack of cards with wild geese flying in a V-shape on the back of them. The engine finally started to roar. The way they do when they're warmed up on cold December mornings.

We took the byroad again and ran parallel with the new bypass for a few hundred yards. A steady stream of lights shot out along it like falling stars. Bumper leaned over between the seats. He was back on form now he knew he didn't have to drive. He was smoking again. Ash fell on my shoulders but I was too busy trying to keep a line between what seemed to be two constantly converging ditches to do anything about it.

—I enjoy these oul jaunts. Going out for a spin and having a few pints. It makes life more interesting.

—We put a lot of fucking miles on the clock today just to get a few pints.

—In fairness now, give us a bit of credit for using this.

He tried to tap his head but his finger missed in the dark and hit off the back of my seat. He put his finger in his mouth then. It made him sound like he was talking under water.

—I just had to see a few heads like. To find out what all this crack is about.

—Did you?

—Yeah.

—Well.

—You were saying I was wasting our time, you were fucking implying it.

I held my breath. Bumper's voice was a lot calmer when he eventually spoke again.

—Your brother and Noelie and a couple of other lads were in a gang together. They were involved in some sort of a scam and it cut across another crowd. Heavy hoors. From over in Abbeytown. I don't have their names but I have names to get their names. We'll sort them.

Abbeytown was thirty miles from Rathbawn. In a different county. On a different train line to Dublin. It seemed like cheating Johnny to come that far to kill him. It seemed like cheating me to bring me this far to find my brother had been a robber.

—What sort of stuff were Johnny and Beetlejuice at?

—You know all those empty houses in the Park. The minute anyone moved out of one they took everything out of it. Stairs, range, bath, they even took the light switches off the wall. They did a great job. Fuck.

Bumper's hands flew out over my shoulder and caught hold of the wheel. The car nearly spun into the ditch.

—Fuck's sake Paul, in the name of Jesus turn the car round. It's a bastarding checkpoint.

Three squads with dimmed lights were parked up ahead. Just before a grove of trees that hung over a patch of road and kept it dark even in daylight. Two men with torches in their hands did little jumps up and down in the middle of the road to keep themselves warm.

—Fucking swing the car round.

Bumper had one of those kung fu weapons made out of a chain and a bar in his hand. I knew he had a hatchet and a butcher's knife in his coat as well. I reversed slowly and hoped the shades would reckon we had just taken a wrong turn. The torchlight shone in our direction. Two squad engines were switched on. I swung the car round and put the pedal to the metal. Bumper slammed against the back of my seat. The non-chucks flew out of his hand and clattered off the dashboard before disappearing into the dark recesses of the car floor.

I lost control of the Opel when we came round a bend under a railway bridge. We spun across the road. I put my hands over my head. Bumper cursed. We both got ready for the inevitable big wallop from something or other.

It never happened. The car stopped in the middle of the road. The inside seemed to be moving. I puked my ring up on the steering wheel. Some of it splashed back on my clothes. Bumper dragged me out of the car. The lights of the squads arced around the corner and fell on our backs. Like sentry-tower lights from *The Great Escape* as the Brits try to get under the barbed wire.

More barbed wire as Bumper bundled me over a fence and into a field. I landed in a ditch and my chin jolted against the ground. Bumper grabbed hold of me under the arm and dragged me along after him. On my knees. For the first few yards. When I stood up he kept dragging me. The cops shone torches into the field and shouted after us in a half-hearted way.

—There's no point in running, lads. We know who ye are.

But we knew that they didn't and that some young fella in Rathbawn who had a name of knackering Opels would be getting a wake-up call in a few hours.

We fell over the dark for what might have been a couple of hours and got diagonally back to somewhere on the road. Beside a small, red, galvanized shed across the road from a pub with two old-fashioned petrol pumps standing in front of it. The pumps were a greeny colour and the petrol was a brand no one had used these years.

You only cop how useful and warm houses are when you try and sleep without one. Bumper rolled fags all night and told me stories about his relations. One uncle slept rough for years and caught gangrene, which meant both his legs had to be amputated. I felt unhealthy twinges in my shins and knees as Bumper's voice started to wind down.

He told me he wanted to be a prison officer when he was young. I told him I wanted to be an astronaut. He didn't answer. I said it again. There was silence except for the noise of Bumper's snores. And the sound of little creatures scraping away in the corner of the shed.

Another night of trying to blame myself for what had happened to Lydia. My oldies but goldies. I worked a bit too much. I drank a bit too much. There must have been some gap on the track of our lives to shunt her so far off the rails.

But I know that is basically a load of balls.

People blame themselves for selfish reasons. They can bear the fact that they are flawed themselves. Because that can be altered. What they can't bear is that life has unfairness running through it like the San Andreas Fault. The love you take is not equal to the love you make. Not in the end. Not at the start. Life is not the secondary-school science experiment where a piece of elastic gets stretched in direct proportion to the weights suspended from it.

When I heard first about Bishop Casey and Annie Murphy I just thought I hadn't been listening to the *News* properly. Some facts don't register the first time around. Or the second.

Lydia couldn't speak three words to me. She couldn't look at Kaya. I wouldn't know where she was for hours at a time. In hindsight it looks obvious. Does it? I thought she had post-natal thingumajig. Maybe she did. Maybe that started her off. Maybe it is my fault after all. Mine and Kaya's.

Some days I thought she was just bored. With me. Or depressed because that spring was a miserable and damp one. She stared, pale-faced, off into the sky the day we visited Alton Towers.

I sacked three assistant managers in a row for stealing from the till. When I told O'Neill he wondered out loud if my judgement was getting weak. He said you can always tell the kind of sketch who'll rip you off.

—Just by looking at their eyes, Paul, it's easy done.

One night I nearly even rang Mam.

—You're a fool to yourself.

I always hated that phrase. There's a certain type of hoor loves saying it. They actually mean:

—Wouldn't you be far better off if you were a miserable, mangy, mean-spirited mink like me?

Only. Only. Only one morning Vinnie said it to me. I was so mad I wanted to fire him. And then I thought, what's fucking wrong with you this weather? What has you getting like this? With Vinnie.

A new mob had started drinking in the lounge. Loud Londoners. Except for their leader. Gangs of people are like gangs of lemmings. They need someone in front so they know where they're going.

This lemon was called Sean. A Dub with a rugby inter-national's accent. He carried a mobile phone around and walked the lounge of my pub like it was the kitchen of his house. His feet were up on the counter when I walked in this day.

—Sonny, get your fucking feet down off the fucking counter.

—You what?

—Listen, Paddy. You heard me too fucking well. Down with the spawgs, like a good lad.

The blue deck shoes inched off the counter. Even the fuck's feet were suntanned. Or solarium-tanned. Or he could have got the colour from a hard day's work on the bog. The feet came down. Slowly. He said something under his breath to the lad beside him. He got a giggle in response. A subordinate's giggle. I would have let it go but that day I was like a bull for some reason I still didn't know.

—Right, you bollocks. Out of this pub the lot of ye. Come on, savvy? Do you want me to put up a big red neon sign on it for ye? Get to fuck out of my pub.

They shuffled around with Rizlas and grudgingly removed expensive jackets from the backs of chairs. Sean would have liked to cut my throat just then. But the lounge was full of my regulars. And the football team had come in from the public bar. Sean wasn't a hard man. Not the way it says in the manual. The original manual. I walked out from behind the counter. Lydia followed me. Vinnie came as well. Lydia spoke first.

—I'm sorry about this, Sean.

He smiled. I pushed him out the door after the rest of the gang.

—I'm sorry too. Have a nice day . . . you cunt.

The regulars started clapping the second the door closed. A funny sort of relief was in the air. But I don't recommend slaying other people's dragons for them. It's not majorly satisfying.

—You wanker, Lydia seemed to whisper as I walked past her.

I couldn't imagine why she would have, so half a second later I decided she hadn't. Now I know she must have. Or maybe I did mishear her. She mightn't have said anything at all. She might have been muttering to herself. The old significance airbrush again. Beware.

Quid coins rattled in the lounge. Another big win on the Trivia Super Challenge machine. I'd have to get the company to send a different make. The questions were way too easy at the moment.

Eight

Iowa, Ohio, Idaho

It was early in the morning. We were eight miles from Rathbawn on a long, straight stretch of road. The cars we did see were ploughing along at a great clip. We didn't say it but the reason we kept walking was because there was no point in waiting around for a lift. Neither of us knew anyone who'd be driving anywhere at this hour of the morning. Not unpursued anyways.

We hadn't even bothered to thumb the lorry that pulled up beside us. A huge painting of a cow with giant red italic writing underneath it adorned the front. *The Brown Bull of Ballytoghert.*

—Mornin', buddies, I reckon y'all could be doing with a ride, said the Bull himself.

—You're fucking right there.

The Brown Bull's words came out

as quickly as the bits of miles flying by on the hyperactive speedometer.

—I gotta keep talking to keep myself awake. Done brought this rig across from Germany and now I'm a-heading to my old homestead out West.

The spiel got us all the way to Rathbawn. It was mainly on his chosen subject.

—The foxy ladies I done met on my travels, good buddies.

He kept winking and jerking his thumb back in the direction of a stringy hammock behind the seats. Two little white pillows rested at the top end of it. Any time me or Bumper tried to talk, the Brown Bull sang along with those twanging sounds moseying out of the tape deck.

He dropped us off in Green Street and turned for the west. Heading out for the prairie country.

—See y'around, good buddies.

—And yourself, you son of a bitch.

A four-foot-high stack of newspapers sat outside McDonnell's Newsagents. Bound with thin string tight enough to cut the fingers off anyone who fancied prising a paper from the pile. Bumper lacerated the string with a knife.

—The *Sun* or the *Star*?

Next thing we knew Ozzie Small was coming round the corner with his fists swinging. In such a temper he didn't even know who was there.

—Fuck off, fuck off, now keep away from those papers. Robbers.

Bumper raised the knife to him.

—What's wrong with you, you mad bastard?

Ozzie held a carton of milk in either fist. Bumper swung the knife and sliced one of them into two bits. Milk splashed all over Ozzie's trousers and the bottom half of the empty carton bounced against the window of McDonnell's. Ozzie hugged the other carton protectively to his chest and looked sadly at the empty container half in his hand and the puddle of milk at his feet.

—That's Missus Callaghan's milk, boys. What am I going to do now?

Bumper tucked the knife back into his coat. He got it tough not to laugh into Ozzie's face. Ozzie was whining. It was fairly fucking pathetic.

—That fucking Jody thinks he's a smart boy but I'm smarter than he is. You have to be up early to catch out Ozzie Small. I'm here all morning waiting for the shops to open. I have Missus Callaghan's milk and he doesn't.

—You *had* Missus Callaghan's milk.

Bumper picked up a sheaf of papers and threw them into the gutter. The pages scattered in several directions. Like black-backed gulls breaking out of formation.

—I still have one carton.

Ozzie ignored us completely as he searched through the piles of paper for the *Irish Independent* that could be brought intact to Missus Callaghan at half ten. We left him there. Singing and trying to put some order on a heap of defunct rain forest.

—Do you want to come for a healer?

I shook my head.

Kaya's and Mam's sleeping breath filled the house. I wondered when I'd last slept like that. Without the block running across the middle of my mind. I wondered a lot of things. It kills the hours. They'd die anyways but it's nice to think you're shooting at them yourself.

I wondered if I still blamed Mam. Though I knew it wasn't her fault. It had never been her fault. But admitting the futility of arguments is the hardest thing to do. If you admit you're wrong, it's all been pointless. All that hatred and in the long run you were as well off pulling your wire.

I don't hate Mam. I don't think I ever did. I just think I thought I did. I think. She must have done something to drive him away. Because for a long time he kept coming back.

Those were the worst times of all. Unreal quiet as we waited for the explosion. Then the sound of him piling stuff into this battered blue suitcase someone had bought them for the wedding. The sight of him dragging the suitcase out the front door and fucking it over the gate into the road. The sound of him slamming the gate like he was trying to break it. The sight of the suitcase springing open when it hit the road and exposing my oul fella's socks, jocks and vests to the world. And the sight and sound of the neighbours laughing.

I used think it was Mam they were laughing at because they kept their faces straight until he had stomped out of earshot.

He never hit her. She told me that. But he broke tables, windows, chairs and two little china milkmaids that sat on the kitchen mantelpiece. Liz used play with them. She made them hold imaginary conversations with each other. Missus and Miss.

But it wasn't him I blamed. Even though I know he felt well shot of the gang of us. He didn't have great time for Mam or me or Johnny or anyone else who wasn't the Joe Kelly who the *Champion* cutting said had married Nuala Briody with nuptial mass and Papal Blessing in June 1958.

Who says your father has to like you, who? Why should he? Why should he like you any more than any of the other people he met in his life? Should he like just because you're his son? Who says he has to? Your mother at least has to do the Stations of the Cross with you for nine months. But your oul fella doesn't even have to know you're born. Some don't. So why should he give a toss for you if he doesn't want to? Where does it say he has to?

We got bulletins about him. Sometimes twice a year. Sometimes less. From people who'd met him in Boston. Never one word from himself. Just these communiqués from people who'd worked on the buildings with him.

—He's making sure to wear a hard hat the whole time, Missus Kelly. Because the heat would drive you mad. It'd boil your brains, so it would, so you can't go around bareheaded.

Mam was in Quinnsworth one day when she got stuck with a high number at the meat counter and a man started chatting her.

—I was on the skite with him on his last night in Boston and he told me that the next day he was packing in the stone cladding and heading out west. Iowa, I'm nearly sure he said.

Or Ohio. Or Idaho. One of the three places anyways, the man at the meat counter was definite.

—Iowa, Ohio, Idaho.

Like the refrain of a hit for a Fifties doo-wop group. Or a black-and-white movie musical number with the young Astaire buck tapping his feet in time to the chant.

—Iowa, Ohio, Idaho.

I was still thinking about Fred Astaire poncing around a giant sound-stage when I got up to watch *Coronation Street*. Just like old times. Me, Mam and Kaya sitting there. Nobody saying anything. The only sound the hum of migraines being nursed and revenge for unspecified wrongs being considered. Mam and Kaya went out to the kitchen during the ad break. They didn't come back for the second half. Mam's voice sniped in the sitting-room door.

—Paul, Gerry's here to see you.

Gerry? Clinger. With a copy of *Shoot* under his arm. White in the face still from his days in hospital. The wailing trumpet at the end of the *Street* put him off his stroke for a few seconds. Did I look as old as he did?

—I brought you down a *Shoot*. There's an interview with Roy in it.

But neither of us were on for talking about football this evening.

—I'm sorry I didn't go down to see you in hospital. I was sort of a bit shook myself.

—It's all right. I don't know what I was at chasing after yer man. I must be fucking mad and me a father now.

—. . .

—Being a father and all that, you know, I couldn't afford to get killed.

—You're fucking joking me.

—Nah. Bernie popped last night. It was fucking gas. Eddie was after coming in to bring me home and Bernie was in the car with him. Didn't she go into labour on her way to the hospital.

A smile came up at the back of his eyes. Like a powerful fog lamp on a misty night. I thought of Bernie's thin white ankles. And the way her body got lost in that big parka. Fourteen hours Lydia was in it. Several times she fucked and blinded at me and told me she'd kill me for planting her like this.

And then Kaya out of it. They look too fucking small. They make you think of what a miracle it was you ever survived. They make all the other bits of your life seem a bit of a come-down after the hearing of that first cry. It can't be explained because it's only a split second. The words are letting me down again. What can you say about it that has anything to do with what it's really like?

—Congratulations, Clinger.

—Thanks.

—No, seriously, I do mean it. Congratulations. In all seriousness. It fucking means something.

—Thanks.

It was a boy. They were going calling it Eddie.

—After Eddie.

Clinger wanted to know about kids. When they started walking. When they started talking. When they started teething and if that was as bad as it was made out to be. I said it wasn't. It was a lot worse. I told him they'd have a better chance of getting a house off the Council now.

—D'you know, I never even thought of that.

I knew. I poured two glasses of poitin. From the Sanor Raspberry Cordial bottle Beetlejuice had left on our sitting-room floor. When he had existed and young Eddie had not. Clink.

—To fatherhood.

—To fatherhood.

—You know, Clinger, a man can be a father to millions but he can be a dad to only a few.

—What?

—Nothing.

It started to make gentle rain outside. The kids were caught. Perplexed. Unsure whether it was wet enough to go inside or dry enough to stay outside. Clinger joined me at the window. He twisted a sleeper nervously around in his ear.

The phone rang. I knew it was for me. The way sometimes you know what the next song is going to be on the radio a couple of seconds before it starts. Mam called my name.

—I better head then, Paul.

—Yeah, I'll see you again.

I was going to tell him I wouldn't be at home tomorrow. I was going to make up some excuse. But I didn't. Because I had a feeling I really would be gone somewhere. It seemed fairer to let him turn up and hear the news from Mam who, everyone knew, always told the truth.

The receiver was off the hook in the hall. I walked past it and into the kitchen where Mam pretended to dry an almost desiccated plate.

—Who is it?

—A girl. She says she's a friend but she wouldn't give me her name.

—Oh.

Mam's face splintered into a reluctant smile. Kaya in the back yard carried a sod of brown turf in each hand and looked at them.

—Do you want a cup of tea?

—I'd murder one.

—I'll bring it out to you.

Whoever had called had gone away from the phone. There was no sound at the other end of the line. But the silence sounded familiar. I heard the caller walking across a room. Somewhere. They picked up the receiver. I stayed silent. I wanted them to speak first. They were the one who'd called after all.

—Hello.

—Kerrie.

Pearl-divers can hold their breath under water for two minutes. I sounded like one who'd done it for three and a half and just come up to tell the boatmen he'd nearly had his goolies bitten off by a shark.

—Hiya, Paul.

Her voice sounded like she was greeting me at the breakfast table. A more normal, TV sit-com table than the one which usually stood between us. With me away, she wouldn't stay in the pub. I knew that. She'd sleep every night in the squat five floors up on the Clifton Estate that Kiwi students used for short stays. Kerrie had been kipping there for a record span now. I felt angry for getting a pang at the thought of her sleeping apart from me.

—How the fuck did you get this number? I never gave it out to anyone.

Kerrie's nervous laughter sent a small crackle down the line. A jumpy erotic sound that crossed the Irish Sea instantaneously.

—It's a really long story, Paul.

Rilly. Maybe she sounded really different on the phone. Some people do. Or maybe the accent sounded so strange because I'd heard nothing only people speaking the same as each other the last few days.

—Kel, tell me how you found the number. I like stories.

—Just like Kaya. How's she been? Is she happy and everything? Can I speak to her?

—She's great. They're making a great fuss of her. She's gone to bed now. How'd you get the number?

—Well. First we rang International Enquiries but they said the number was ex-directory and they wouldn't give it to us. Then Vinnie remembered the time one of your neighbours came into the pub. That guy who lived next door to you. Paddy something. He drinks in the Admiral Nelson. So we went down there. His wife was behind the bar and she said he'd be in at six for a pint, so me and Vinnie waited for a couple of hours until he came in. He didn't know your mum's number but he rang his own mum and she told him.

Herself and Vinnie. I should have asked her who was running the fucking pub. But I didn't.

—Jesus, Kerrie, you shouldn't have gone to all that trouble.

—It was . . . no hass.

A gurgle was what came down the line this time. Definitely. A gurgle is the only way to describe it.

—So, Paul, are you OK? You're not letting things get on top of you?

One night I woke up to find Kerrie rubbing cold sweat off my back with a sopping towel.

—I'm OK. I'm a bit tired but. Honestly, Kel, are you all right? I'm sorry about having to leave so fast and I'm sorry about being so awful the day before. No. Seriously this time.

She went to say something straight away in reply but then it caught in the back of her throat and was gone for ever.

—So, I hope the funeral went OK. I mean, all the arrangements came off proper. It must have been a very sad occasion for everyone in the family.

—It was but it was OK as funerals go. There haven't been any problems in the pub? O'Neill hasn't been giving out about me going away or anything?

A key turned in the lock. Tracey switched on the hall light and slung her scarf across a hook above the hall table. Dank would have been a good word for the look she gave me.

—No. There's been no problems. Vinnie's handling everything OK. Ammm . . . Oh, I don't know. When are you going to be back?

—Jesus, it's difficult . . . Ahhh . . . soon maybe . . . Yeah, you know, do you miss me?

—Of course I do. I miss you a lot. I wish you were back here. Honestly I do. Go on, tell me you miss me too.

—I . . . Ah . . . I miss you too. No, I do. I miss you a good bit. Tell Vinnie I was asking for him and to keep his pecker up. I'll give ye a ring in a few days. 'Bye.

—'Bye, 'bye, 'bye, see you, pet.

Pit. She always ended phone calls with that machine-gun 'bye 'bye 'bye. As if there was so much more she could have said, so all the remaining energy had to be pumped into the farewell.

I tried to recover the sound of her voice from the air. The tone of it. It had changed three or four times over those few minutes. The different modes. They probably mean nothing. It's just the way people talk. It's like trying to decipher those signs the mad Celts left on the standing stones. Ogham. It'd be a pure cinch if you knew the language.

All I was asking for was a handbook to tell me what people were saying. Exactly what they were saying. Kerrie. What? A couple of pints or I wouldn't be able to sleep on it.

Joe turned and polished his set of the brass monkeys who see, hear and speak no evil when Bumper walked into

Donoghue's. Bumper didn't look at him. He handed me a Rothman's packet.

—There's a name and address written on that, a girl in Cordrum. The word is she knows who killed the boys. You should go over and see her tomorrow. I can't do it, I'm known around there and she'd run a million miles to get away from one of my smiles. See you tomorrow. Hey, Mr Donoghue, do their balls really freeze off when it gets cold?

Bumper's slab-like lettering had punched two holes in the back of the fag box.

—Theresa Lawrence, 42 Bobby Sands Villas. PS: She's a knacker.

Two shaggy piebald horses with blue ropes dangling from their necks cantered down Bakers Lane as I took both sides of it on the way home. Barney Devine drove past in a battered Cortina with so little thread on the tyres it was a miracle the wheels went round. I stood still and listened to the sound of night in the Park. One siren. Two sirens.

Nine

If Mr Skill Could See Me Now

Someone was attacking me in my dream. I was trapped. Cornered. By two men with guns. I made a big effort and wrenched myself out of sleep. It was the only way to escape. Wake up.

I was sure I was awake. But I was still being attacked. Someone was hitting me in the face. I threw my hands out in front of my face and rolled on to my side. I don't have the foggiest notion what use that would have been if someone had been attacking me. It didn't have much effect on Kaya. She just decided to pull my hair instead of poking her fingers into my face.

—Dad, Dad, wake up, Dad.

That London accent again. I picked her up and held her in the air for a few seconds. This usually made her giggle. But she wasn't on for the giggling game this morning. She was serious. Seriously serious. Her usual

I'm-so-serious face looked so out of place it made people laugh. But this was a different face.

—Dad, am I going to die?

—No, you're not.

—But you said that everyone's got to.

—When?

—You did. You said it.

Vague memories of a conversation something like this a few months back. But no memory of what I said. I think I called in Kerrie to rescue me and went downstairs for a pint.

—Dad.

The word was pitched halfway between a complaint and an encouragement and hedged all the way round with a question.

—Well, you are. But not for ages. Not for a hundred years, really.

—I don't want to die.

—Stop being silly. Everyone has to die but you're not going to for ages and ages.

I asked her why she was so worried about dying all of a sudden. I wasn't that interested in her answer. I just had to talk to show her I was in control. Because most of Kaya's queries ended up with questions about Lydia. Questions I pretended I'd never have to answer.

—Granny Kelly says that when you die you float around up in the sky.

Fuck's sake, Mam, make it difficult for me, why don't you?

—You don't really. It's just like going asleep.

—Going to sleep.

Kaya repeated Kerrie's automatic correction.

—You don't float around up in the sky. Unless you're a balloon.

—Or Twinkle, Twinkle, Little Star, Kaya muttered to herself.

—There's one that goes 'Twinkle, Twinkle, Little Bat'.
Kaya giggled when I said that. I was encouraged.

—It's in a book about a girl called Alice.

—Who the fuck is Alice?

She bowed her head immediately to inspect phantom specks of dust on her toddler-issue Nikes even though she knew I wouldn't say anything to her. Her head came back above the surface in a couple of seconds. She looked me bang in the middle of the eye. Her eyes caught the light in a way that reflected me in the centre of her pupils. Drowning in them.

—Granny Kelly says that angels float around above the clouds.

—They fly around. Sure you know about angels, don't you? Good girl. Angels are good.

If I told her she had a guardian angel, she'd probably look over her shoulder expecting to see a hard chaw wearing a red Kangol hat.

—You said Mum is an angel.

—She is.

Please don't talk about your mum like a good girl.

—Does Mum have to float around all day then?

Socratic discourse, as Kerrie says when me and Vinnie are in the middle of an argument about whose turn it is to go down and buy the kebabs after closing time.

—I don't know. Maybe she does. It's very nice up there in Heaven. Flying around.

—I don't want to go to Heaven. I don't want to float around. I want to stay here.

I sat her on my knee and told a couple of jokes to try and cheer her up so she wouldn't guess I was ten times more scared than she was.

—Are you scared now, Goldilocks?

—Nah. Were you ever scared of anything?

—No, I was never scared of anybody, Goldilocks.

—Don't call me Goldilocks, Dad, it's a sad name.

I swung the wardrobe doors wide open and threw my clothes on to the bed quick as I could. I had to avoid looking at the bottom of the wardrobe. Always reminders of Johnny there. Odd socks, discoloured boxer shorts, a floral dicky-bow with long-since dehydrated Guinness discolouring half of it. I swiped the clothes out at top speed and took the risk of creasing them.

Four pairs of boxers got rejected before I came to a pair with Betty Boop pouting as hearts flew out of her mouth. Lydia presented them to me at our last Christmas dinner together. In a Mexican restaurant in Norwood that turned festive and traditional every 25 December. She produced them from her handbag and tossed them across the table to me. They upset a candle. The brown singe mark was still at the crotch.

Bumper was waiting at the top of Bakers Lane. In a car with the registration number painted on the plate and three days' tax cover on the front window. He jumped out of the car when he saw me coming.

—You should fucking be in fucking Cordrum.

—Fuck off. I didn't get time to go yet.

—Ah, now, fuck's sake.

He thumped the front wing of the car. Little clusters of rust flakes fell into the rainbow puddle of oil beside him.

—I'll go in a bit, Bumper.

—Why can't you go now? You're not shitting it, are you? Are you serious?

It made me feel guilty that there was more sorrow than temper in the sound of his voice.

—I am serious.

—You're not really.

—I am. God's honest truth.

—Jump in then. I'll leave you over to Cordrum. But you can make your own fucking way back. And when I say serious I mean this is more important than anything else.

It was the quietest journey we ever made together. And the slowest. Bumper said he couldn't put the car over thirty or black smoke would start puffing out of the engine. He'd robbed it from Eddie Clyne's scrapyard.

—That Alsatian loves me.

Bumper turned the car four hundred yards before the road into Bobby Sands Villas.

—You know if I could leave you up I would. You know that.

I knew that. Number 42 was on top of a hill. A load of caravans were parked on a further slope above it. Washing hung out on thin lines in front of them and a gang of women and kids milled around. The hedge outside Number 42 was overgrown but there was neat, new white paint on the front wall. The gate was open and the garden small enough for two paces to bring me to the front doorstep. I rang the bell and banged on the front door to make sure.

A small, black-haired woman answered the door with a kid either side of her. Her bare brown legs made a swishing noise as she walked down the short hall. The beauty spots on either side of her nose were geometrically balanced.

—I'm looking for Theresa Lawrence.

—Why are you looking for Theresa Lawrence?

—A friend of mine knows her. He told me to look her up if I was ever on this patch.

Pure falseness and dishonesty dripped off my tongue. I hoped the woman would put this down to nervousness. Because I had plenty of it.

—What friend was this? I don't believe you.

Her eyes glazed with a mixture of fright and anger. One

eye green, the other blue in the top half and brown in the bottom half.

—My name's Paul Kelly. I'm from Rathbawn. I'm only home for my brother Johnny's funeral. I'm in England these past eight years.

She spoke in a lullaby sort of a way.

—Are you Johnny's brother, the pub man?

—I am. I was home for the funeral and someone said he mentioned your name. I'm sorry if I'm hassling you, I only want to meet some of the people that knew him.

—I'm Theresa Lawrence. I'm sorry for leaving you on the step but I thought you might be a cop or some sort of a spy.

When I sat at the kitchen table of Number 42 Bobby Sands Villas with Theresa Lawrence, I felt fully jealous of my younger brother for the first time in my life. He didn't seem like a younger brother any more. More like a rival. Or a mystery whose solving would show I hadn't even known what I was investigating.

I didn't know the man at all.

—Someone told me you might know who killed Johnny. Or why he was killed.

—I don't have a clue who killed him or why. I just wish they never done it.

She looked into her cup of tea and lowered her voice when she told me herself and Johnny had a thing going. Those were the words she used. She didn't know much about him all the same, she said. He drew back if questions got asked. But once a week he'd land over to Cordrum and spend the day with her. She never went to Rathbawn with him.

—He said his family would have a fit if they knew he was going out with a traveller woman.

I thought of Uncle Jimmy and Johnny Cash and said nothing. I really did bite my lip and tasted a small drop of blood on my tongue before I took another mouthful of tea.

—I'm as sorry that he's dead. It seems to happen me.

Her husband got stabbed to death after a wedding in Dundalk a couple of years before. His name was Lawrence as well. She explained there was a curse on her and all belonging to her. Then she told me to mind the house while she went to the shops to buy something for the tea. I listened to the rain pelting down when she was away and watched the telly with her two boys. Simon was Kaya's age. Tommy was maybe a year older. But they seemed to have more on the clock. They were wary.

Theresa told me she watched cooking programmes the whole time on the telly. They seemed more interesting and more use than anything else. She emptied steak in a pepper sauce, garlic potatoes and mushrooms on to my plate. A bottle of red wine kept her company when she returned from the kitchen. She beheaded it with one impressive sweep of a dilapidated corkscrew. Pound and penny signs and question marks must have come up in my eyes.

—It's seldom I'll have anyone to dinner with Johnny gone. Today would have been his day.

I looked out the window when I finished the grub. A burly man with a red moustache wove a drunken way along the footpath. He stopped in front of Number 42.

—Gyppo, gyp. Gyp, gyp. Gyppo.

Theresa flung herself past me and hammered on the window.

—Cunt, you fucking cunt, fuck off and leave me alone.

The man's eyes locked into hers. He gave her the fingers in the style of a magician producing a white dove from under a cloak and tottered along before he stumbled in the gate of Number 44. Red scrape marks showed on the knuckles of Theresa's left hand when she took it away from the window.

—That cunt is at it since I moved in here. He's a real bastard. Johnny followed him up to his house one evening and kicked him along the footpath. Yer man rolled in under a car. It was fierce crack. He wouldn't come out and Johnny kept roaring and trying to get a right skelp at him. It put manners on the boyo for a while. Johnny was a fucking hard man.

She smiled. I was being invited to feel pride. It was more of a beam than a smile. I looked at my own feet and thought of the sound of cogs on the way up to the Dispensary when Johnny kicked with a tiny football boot. I don't know what I thought I'd do when I heard the knock on the door. But I loitered in the hall behind Theresa when she went to answer it.

A lad my own age with black beard crouching protectively around the edges of his face handed a rolled-up newspaper to Theresa. He half bowed and raised one of his eyebrows when he saw me.

—Thanks for the lend of the paper, Iack.

Theresa kept watching as he shuffled slowly towards the caravans. She took a quick wet breath in through her nostrils before she shut the door.

—If we couldn't import friends, we'd have none in this place.

Bobby Sands Villas was better off than Colmcille Park. It had MTV on the cable. It helped me and Theresa and Tommy and Simon communicate wordlessly by staring at hours of hair lacquer, powder and paint and exchanging nods and shrugs at the funny or sad bits. Theresa disappeared periodically and returned with cans of lager. She kept apologizing for only buying one bottle of wine. She told me she'd noticed how whenever someone sat down to eat in *EastEnders* there was a bottle of wine at the table.

—Johnny knew a lot about wine.

I don't know whether she was obsessed with Johnny or whether she was seeking safety on the one acre of common ground. But every time her voice got into its full flow like a nervy skylark Johnny's name was there to come between us and remind us we weren't just two strangers in the night watching MTV together for the sake of company.

—I'm scared to fall asleep since he died. The doc has me on Librium but it's no good. I still feel like a fraidy cat. What I'd love to get hold of is that Prozac stuff, they reckon it makes you happy for ever. It's supposed to be mighty.

Theresa took off her shoes and curled her legs back under herself when she had Tommy and Simon tucked into bed.

—Did Johnny ever say anything about our mother?

—He said she doted on him. He said if she had her way she'd make him build a house in her back garden and come up to him every morning to bring him tea and toast and collect his dirty washing.

An unspoken cruelty somewhere in the comment begged the next question.

—Did he say anything about me ever?

—Hardly. If he got footless drunk, he'd start laughing and call you Mr Skill. 'I wonder what Mr Skill is at today,' 'I wonder is Mr Skill ever going to come home,' 'If Mr Skill could see me now.'

Mr Skill. Imaginary super-hero and secret agent of our childhood. He roamed the length and breadth of Colmcille Park, doing battle with Tegratol, the most powerful villain in the universe, named after the tablets Uncle Jimmy took to combat the epilepsy we dreaded inheriting.

—So, Mr Skill, we meet again.

—Tegratol, I should have known you'd be mixed up in this somewhere.

Theresa was on another scurry to the fridge when I realized we'd met before. And that I'd thought about that meeting for a long time after.

At Courtown, me and Johnny did what all ten- and eight-year-olds at the seaside do. We got into a gang with other scrawny adventurers. Mr Skill may have been involved but that is one thing I don't remember. The other castle builders and shell collectors bled away as the light did until there were just four of us left. Myself, Johnny, a red-haired local lad named Eoghan who held a crab captive in a green sandbucket with fancy turrets and a small girl who hadn't spoken two words all day. All she did was follow every move faithfully. And fling shards of delighted laughter that shattered the cooling air as we sat down at the edge of the sea and let the tide wash past us. We asked her name when the sun went behind its last cloud of the day.

—I'm not telling you.

—What's your name? You know ours.

—I'm told not to tell anyone my name.

—Well, then, you're not our friend.

We turned on our heels and walked back for dry land. The girl scampered after us at top speed on small brown, bruise-mottled legs.

—Theresa Lawrence, Theresa Lawrence, Theresa Lawrence.

She didn't ask for money till the goodbyes had been said.

—Have you got some money for us? You must have some.

We told her we didn't but she kept following us up the beach. There was something strange about the grip she had on my arm. I thought then it was the Chinese burn but I know now it might have been something to do with fear.

—Ye have money. Just give us a few pence for sweets.

Her voice got higher and faster and shriller as we drew nearer to the hot tarmac and Ford Cortinas. Eoghan looked dolefully down at the crab and poked him in the hope of extracting a reaction. There wasn't and there wouldn't be one.

—Could ye not get money? Could ye not ask yere parents to give ye money and say it's for yereselves and give me some of it?

We were twenty yards away from the cars when the old woman with the pouched skin and the white hair piled up in a bun stepped across us and grabbed Theresa by the shoulder.

—You. Get in home.

—I'm sorry, Granny. I was playing with these boys.

Granny stopped to blow her nose. Her eyes watered with hay fever. She caught the snot expertly between thumb and forefinger and flicked it into the sky. She came close enough for the smell of drink and warm air to wrap a necklace round my face.

—Have you any money, young fella? Tell the truth now and shame the divil, just a few pence for a sup of milk for the babby.

—No, I don't, I said because I didn't.

Her granny pulled Theresa along by the arm. Theresa's feet made inconsistent contact with the ground till she shook free and walked full pelt to their caravan. Each of them seemed to harbour a secret sulk against the other. Then, like it always did, it started to rain. But I forget what kind of rain it was or what weight it carried. I remember the parti-coloured eyes and the beauty spots perfectly aligned on either side of a face bunched up from working out angles. All those years ago. I wondered if Johnny had remembered.

Maybe my memory came in a dream because I suddenly seemed to wake and Theresa Lawrence's arms were around me and my mouth was filled with the pink taste of hers before she pulled away and grinned.

—I don't know what you think, Mr Skill, but I think it's gone a bit late for you to try and save the world anywhere else tonight.

Ten

And Information Made Him Fat

The rain tried to knock down the house. It might have been the rain from the flood that was going to end it all. A high wind joined in. Twice glass shattered out in the night.

Most of the time I didn't hear the wind or the rain. All I heard was Theresa Lawrence and her wild calmness. Choking and panting and spitting in my ear from below me in the dark. Breathing through her nose as she rose above me and the outline of flapping clothes in the back yard jumped across her body in a shadow-play.

—Again, come on.

Her teeth and her lips unevenly grazing the side of my head and my ears as we looked over each other's shoulders at the darkness, the walls and the windows.

—Come on, again.

Pulling and dragging and kneading to keep it going when it seemed impossible. Stumbling up and down a rackety bed with broken springs, tangling in the duvet, slipping across discarded clothes and pausing at odd skew-ways angles with our mouths licking each other's openings and our noses sunk deep in an odour of sweat and spunk and juice. Waiting. Breathing.

—You're not going to get a fucking heart attack, are you?

I felt out of myself in the jangling and creaking bed. Like I hadn't since Lydia died. I wasn't looking at myself any more. I was just doing. And when the thoughts and the questions started slithering back across my mind I felt the nip of the rings on Theresa's fingers bringing me back to the dark and the shadows.

—You're not gone asleep, sure you're not?

She had kicked the side of the bed and leaned against the wardrobe when she saw the empty plastic container. The Librium prescription unfurled beside it on the bedside locker. Theresa sat on the edge of the bed with her jeans round her knees. Her white hands shook as they gripped those brown legs.

—Fuck it. I haven't a hope of getting a wink of sleep now.

She grabbed my waist and dragged me down on the bed. Her eyes closed the split second before she wrenched the bedside-lamp plug out of the wall.

The rain spent a lot of its time dripping through holes in the bedroom roof. Splashing into a saucepan positioned accurately under the main waterfall. In the morning there was enough water there to cover a boiling egg. Every metallic report a strange robotic accompaniment to sex.

Listen for the next drop. When I was a nipper I could never work out what was so bad about the dripping-water torture. Surely the one with the electric shocks must be far worse.

174

—Listen to the ponny.

The only words she spoke quietly all night. We didn't talk then. Noises squeezed out of our mouths under pressure but they weren't words. We talked in the morning. When the light arrived. And the wind dropped. And the rain eased and gave way to one of those fakey suns that illuminate the start of a bad day.

When the post slid through the letterbox and collapsed on the rubber mat Theresa threw the duvet on to the floor and stretched like a sharp cat. Some sort of tension seemed to drop from her on to the sheets. Like flakes of rust from one of Eddie's cars. Or stardust. She rolled on to her stomach and hung her tiny feet up in the air.

—Again. Come on. One for the road.

—One for the ride.

Her legs wobbled as she walked out of the bedroom with my white shirt around her. She buttoned it right up to the top. It dropped nearly to her knees. I was putting on a blue denim shirt from the wardrobe when she came back with a cup of tea. Discarded condoms lay on the floor like redundant exclamation marks.

—God, it's good to see one of the Kelly brothers doesn't expect his breakfast in bed. And that's Johnny's shirt.

A shiver crawled down my left side. I asked Theresa to swap shirts with me. But she wouldn't. If she had, I wouldn't have needed to run down to the fridge for a can of lager to make the shaking stop.

Tommy and Simon were chattier this morning. But they still tiptoed around like they'd heard the creepy film music and were waiting for the scary thing to happen. Me and Theresa played Operation with them. Never try to take out a man's funny bones for fifty pounds when you've got the shakes. The buzzer sounded so often I felt like a techno DJ. The two boys bit their fingers to try and stall the laughs. Simon fell across the table when he couldn't hold it in any longer. A small drop of his laugh landed on my cheek. I was glad he smiled back at me.

—Johnny was brilliant at Operation. He could do it with both hands, said Tommy.

Theresa jammed her tongue in her cheek and looked up at the ceiling.

The buck with the black beard landed at twelve to bring the boys over to play at the caravans. He looked at me as if there was someone standing behind me and he didn't like the look of them.

—Theresa, are you sure you're all right, lack?

—I'm grand, Martin, honest I am.

Back in bed she lit up a More and asked me if I could be trusted. I didn't answer. She asked me a second time so I nodded but didn't say anything. I crossed my fingers inside her. The fag sneaked a slight odour of burning sticks on to her breath.

—My brother Robbie now, I'd say he knows who killed Johnny only I wouldn't ask him. It wouldn't do me any good to know.

—He'd know. Are you def on that?

—I'd say he would. Robbie knows things.

—Where would I get him?

—In his house. Or down the Sports Complex playing indoor soccer.

—Where does he live?

—He might tell you nothing. Why should he say anything to you?

—I could tell him you sent me.

—You could. Why do you want to know who killed Johnny?

—Curiosity.

—It killed the cat.

—And information made him fat.

She slapped me lightly across the stomach.

—I'm saying nothing.

I kissed her. She kissed me back.

—Where does Robbie live?

—He lives at Number 17 Cusack Square. You might get him there.

I had my clothes on before I realized what I was doing. And how it looked. Theresa dragged the duvet up around her and lay flat on her back. I had my white shirt on now. She turned her back on me and spoke over her shoulder. Carelessly pegged words. I could take them or I could leave them. That was what I was supposed to think.

—When'll you be coming back?

—In a while.

—You have some cheek. All you wanted was the information. Fat cat.

—He was my brother, I thought ye knew about these sorts of things.

She choked back her first answer and turned around. A tic made those pie eyes jump around. She kicked off the duvet and did that cat stretch again. I realized how long it had been since I thought about how beautiful people can be.

—Well, fuck you then, Mr Skill.

Theresa darted a glance towards the empty pill box and made up some table of odds in her head. A box of Durex Fetherlite stung the tip of my ear as I slammed the door behind me. I heard the framed photos of her dead husband and dead Johnny wobble on the chest of drawers as I walked down the hall.

Martin raised his hand as I passed the other side of the road to the caravans. I thought he was waving at me before a lump of a stone flew past my nose. He banged the heel of his hand against his head in cartoon disappointment and walked back into a caravan through a tunnel of heaped car batteries.

Cusack Square was twenty minutes' walk. I kept looking behind to see if Theresa was following me. She wasn't.

There was no answer when I knocked at the front door of Number 17. I heard talking around the back of the house. Two black greyhounds sat in front of the off-white caravan behind Number 17. They started a whinge when I got near them and scuttled away. The caravan door was wide open but I knocked on it all the same and took a few steps back. The man who came out had a plastic bag under each arm and a blue horse tattooed on his neck. He was the dead-down spit of Theresa Lawrence too.

—Are you looking to buy a duvet, lad?

He made to hand me one of the packages. A young woman and three small kids appeared behind him. I nodded my head.

Robbie Lawrence jumped down from the caravan. One of the greyhounds sidled towards him and tripped over the wire running from the caravan to the back window of the house. I followed Robbie round to the front of the house. I was going to tell him what I was doing here but he said he had more stuff I might be interested in taking off his hands.

Robbie's wife left tea in front of us. The telephone waited expectantly in the hallway so I decided to tell Robbie why I was here before Theresa did and hands moved towards the back pockets of jeans. His wife changed the nappy of a beautiful baby with only four toes on his right foot and pretended not to listen to the conversation. A can of petrol sat beside an open fire overflowing with blazing chunks of wood.

—Go on, you'll buy one of these duvets, lad. I'll give you a great price for one. Or two if it'd be handier.

—Are you Robbie Lawrence? Your sister Theresa told me you'd be able to help me.

The wife looked up. Robbie looked at his feet for a

second. He flexed his shoulder muscles before he drawled. Definitely a drawl.

—What do you want done? I don't know you.

—My name's Paul Kelly. I'm Johnny's brother. Johnny that got killed.

—Oh, shite, said the wife from the other side of the room.

Robbie puffed a thick breath out through his teeth. The tips of his ears turned red. He still said nothing.

—Theresa says you know who killed Johnny.

—That fucking cunt says a lot of things.

—Shut up, Lucy, don't talk about my sister that way. So fucking what?

—I want to know who killed him and why they did it.

Robbie shrugged his shoulders and then flexed them again.

—He was a good lad, yere Johnny, I liked him.

—I liked him too, said Robbie's wife and smiled for the first time.

Robbie emptied his tea into the fire. Purple sparks jumped up the chimney.

—I just want to know who it was that killed him.

—I'll tell you because of who you are. But you're better off not knowing and that's not a word of a lie, boss.

He was leaning to light a butted fag he'd picked up off the floor when he heard the back door being kicked in. Robbie looked at me first. Then he saw I was as surprised as he was. And as frightened. That look cost him a second. He was still in the chair when Bumper arrived and stood over him with a blue metal baseball bat that still had some wood splinters clinging to its head.

—I want a fucking name, Redbreast boy.

—Fuck you, Reilly, and the horse you rode in on.

Bumper swung the bat hard enough to give Robbie's elbow a reminder about manners. Robbie didn't make a sound. He just frantically tried to move his fingers. His eyes moved too. The pupils flitted from one side to the other. They were moving too fast. He was trying to work out what I had to do with this. The memory of the reflection of the washing line across Theresa's body made me speak.

—Leave him alone, Bumper. He was going giving me the name. Before you landed.

Full of faith wasn't how you'd describe Bumper's expression. Robbie breathed out in relief when he found his fingers still in working order. Bumper moved the bat so it lay on top of them. Next thing Lucy was out of her chair and swinging at Bumper with a bread knife that passed just in front of his face and nicked the sleeve of his jacket. Bumper jumped back and hit off the wall. A framed picture of the Arsenal team that won the European Cup Winners Cup crashed down against the side of a broken Super Ser heater. The glass sprinkled in hundreds and thousands across the carpet. The child's nappy came undone. The child rolled on the floor.

Bumper put the smile back on his face. Lucy jabbed a couple more times at his stomach but the bread knife looked a bit of a crap weapon now. Bumper could have knocked her head clean off her shoulders with a decent swing of the bat but he didn't. Robbie moved to leap out of the chair but he didn't. He stayed where he was. I looked at him. He looked at me.

—You touch my husband again and I'll go through you with this.

—Lucy, put down the knife.

—Listen to your husband, he has sense. Sure there's no quarrel here.

—I'll give you the name. I was going to do it. You had no need to make shite out of the back door. I'll give you the name. It's no skin off my balls.

Lucy dropped the bread knife and picked up her child.

Bumper battered the bat against the wall hard enough to leave a permanent dunge.

—Stop it, you stupid fuck, will you. You could have left me to get the name.

I was back watching myself on MTV. Bumper switched the bat from his right hand to his left.

—All right then, Redbreast, spit it out. I haven't got the whole day to be chanting to you. Only for this decent man here I'd batter it out of you, and out of your wife and your baby as well.

—Snoopy Giff. Snoopy Giff killed him, he shot yere Noelie and he killed this man's brother.

—Ah, fuck off.

—Snoopy Giff. I swear it, I fucking swear, Bumper. He's even going around the place telling people he done it.

—Why? Snoopy Giff had nothing to do with my brother. Or with this fella's brother.

—He's in with this mob in Abbeytown. There's some big, big bad fucker involved had it in for the two boys.

Bumper battered the bat into the dunge he'd made. The wall crackled. A mark rippled outwards underneath the wallpaper.

—So who's yon big fucker? Who is he? It's his name I fucking want.

—I don't know. I don't know, honest. No one knows who he is or anything about him only I don't think he's from around the place.

—Do you not know everything that's going on, Redbreast?

—No one knows anything about this boy. Not the cops nor anyone else has a clue about him. I wouldn't tell you a lie, Bumper. All I know is Snoopy Giff is strong-arming for him. I wouldn't tell you a lie, Bumper.

—I know you wouldn't, Redbreast, but I brought the bat just to be on the safe side.

Bumper was driving a blue van this time. The floor was covered with wholesale cartons of cigarettes. This mobile was taxed up to date.

—Snoopy Giff.

—Aye.

—Who is he?

—A scumbag.

—Come on, Bumper. I want the sca.

—He's from Abbeytown. Calls himself Snoopy after some nigger singer called Snoopy Dog Doggy.

—Snoop Doggy Dog. He's a rapper, not a singer.

—All them blacks is the same to me. Young Giff thinks he's the cut of this fella anyways.

—A hard boy?

—A bit of a one. He's all covered with tattoos from when he was in Loughan. He did them with broken glass and ink. Two of my brothers was in there the same time. The ink came out of a bottle with a spider on the front of it.

—So this is the man we're going killing.

—Him for a start. And the big man, whoever he is.

Only it wasn't Snoopy Giff Bumper talked about on the way back to Rathbawn. It was Giff's girlfriend. Maybe not the girlfriend. But a girlfriend.

—Do you remember Bubblicious Doherty, Paul?

I remembered Bubblicious Doherty and her leaving Rathbawn when she was fourteen. I remembered how she got the nickname too. Her oul fella used take her down to the lakeshore and get her to swim in the nip by giving her a packet of Bubblicious. I think even then everyone knew it had to do with more than cheap chewing gum. But no one wanted to think about what.

—She had two kids for Giff. He has kids all over the place. He's some hammer-man, he must have scooby-dooed half of Abbeytown. But he's supposed to be mad keen on Bubblicious.

Bumper stayed talking about Bubblicious. Even when I tried to get him to say more about Snoopy Giff. The man who brought us together. He just kept talking about her and wondering out loud where she lived now. He was still at it when we pulled in to the Diamond, past the kids swinging on ropes round the lampposts.

Six of Bumper's kids were kicking football in the front garden. The grass was as big as them. The leather jacket from Cordrum was wrapped round one little fella. The kids stopped moving when Bumper got to the front wall. The ball stayed abandoned in the centre of the garden while they made a suddenly frozen action replay.

—Mammy was looking for you, Daddy.

—Was she?

An oul fella next door held a hedge-knife and tried to clock who I was. The kids didn't move till Bumper picked up a daughter with curls controlled by reams of thick red ribbon. Ice-pop stains dispersed down the front of her Minnie Mouse T-shirt. He swung her around a couple of times. Gently.

—Who's my favourite girl?

—I am, Daddy.

I winked at her. Bumper left her down when he saw me and grabbed his two boys by the right shoulder. One of them looked ten. The other eight. Their hair was cropped down to the last. The older lad looked longingly over at the stationary football.

—These is my two lads, Noel and Jay. Two hardy fucking little men.

—I'd say they are.

Bumper frowned and signed the other kids to move away from him. He lifted Noel's hands and put them in front of his face. Jay put up a guard. Bumper looked down at me and then over at his neighbour leaning over the hedge.

—Right, lads, box.

They danced around for a few seconds. Jay tried to duck in under Noel's guard but the older boy was too quick for him and rattled the side of his face with a solid clout. Noel kept Jay at arm's length and jabbed. Jay hit Noel into the ribs a couple of times. The man at the hedge turned away after a couple of minutes of this. Bumper grabbed his sons and banged their heads together. The cracking sound went through me.

—I want a proper fucking fight now. I'll give the winner a pound coin and there's no dinner for the loser. I fucking mean it, fight proper or I'll beat the shite out of the two of ye.

He pushed them back in together. Little Jay reacted quickest and slammed his fist against Noel's eye. The way Noel pawed at his eye showed he'd have a severe shiner the next day. Jay ducked in under his arms and caught him a few more belts. His brother's freckled face was scored with knuckle marks. Bumper nodded and smiled as Noel took a step backwards.

—He's a little terrier, isn't he? A great bit of stuff for a lad his size.

Noel stepped back so he could use his reach. A series of thumps rocked Jay's head about like a lobster pot on a turbulent sea. He was driven across the garden and dropped on all fours in front of Bumper. The blood pumping from his nose dripped into his mouth and prevented him from saying something which seemed important to him. Bumper dragged him up off the ground. Jay held his hand up against his nose and tried to remove thick clots of dark blood from each nostril. Bumper made him wipe his hands in the grass.

—Come on, Jay, you can't give up, you have to do something to get him back.

Jay looked at me and I might have done something to stop the fight if he hadn't sprinted at Noel and sent him reeling with a succession of flails. Noel pawed at the previously undamaged eye and then walked back towards his brother. There were no more steps back. And the guards were down. Bumper moved around to the rhythm of the punches and the old neighbour let an odd roar out of him.

—Left, right, hook, jab.

More and more blood came out of Jay's nose. A fountain of it sprang into the air when Noel finally clattered him to the ground in front of Bumper. Bumper walked away from Jay and raised Noel's hand in triumph. I bent down to Jay. I felt there was something I should say to him. He landed a red spit on the concrete path, tottered across the garden and shook hands with Noel. The old man clapped. Bumper handed the boys a quid coin each.

—That was a good hard fight, lads, go in and get yereselves cleaned up.

Bumper copped the meaning of the look I gave him. He always did. Dead wide, the Rob Alls.

—Don't tell me you think there's something wrong with that. Fuck it, unless they know how to fight they'll surely be cowed around here. They have to know how to look after themselves. My oul fella done the same with us and it never done me no harm.

He nodded at the spectator next door.

—Isn't that right, Daddy?

The oul lad nodded back and resumed his interrupted onslaught on the hedge.

The front door reminded me of those Russian dolls who all fit inside each other. A thick plasticky door at the front with a double-glazed door inside it. Another slide-across plasticky door came before the wooden door the house must have been born with.

—You can't be too careful. No one's going to get in my front door unbeknownst to me.

We had to go around the back when Bumper discovered he'd lost the key of the first door. Rubbish was dumped all along the narrow laneway at the back of the house. A couple of rats sat in the middle of the lane and looked unflustered when we walked on by.

—We call them kangaroo rats because they can jump up in the air to bite you. The dogs from the Park wouldn't match the rats from the Diamond.

The hatchet I'd last seen protruding from the counter of the Westerner lay beside a pile of chopped wood in the back yard. I wondered for a moment how Bumper had recovered it. The stupidest wonder ever. All he had to do was go in and say he wanted it back.

His wife was waiting for him in the back kitchen. She looked through me and fucked a frying pan just past his head.

—You fucking wanker, what the fuck do you think you're at?

—Ah, Mary, loveen, what's up with you?

—Yafuckeneejitya.

—Where's the oul dinner?

—The oul dinner is in the young greyhound. The rest of us has ours et. You're three and a half hours late. I had you fucking warned.

She didn't have a lot to spare over five feet but she was tall enough to reach for the next item on the shelf over her head and send it spinning across the kitchen at Bumper. The top flew off the bottle of cooking oil when it hit him. A stream of greasy golden liquid lavaed down the front of his jeans. I waited for the explosion.

—Ah, Mary, I'm sorry, will you not cook a small bit of grub for us, we're pure starved.

—No, I won't. You were told before about being at home in time for the dinner.

—I wasn't even drinking.

—No, you were abroad in Cordrum playing Cowboys and Indians. You may get your food there.

—Could you not heat up something for us, like. You're looking very well today.

—Fuck you.

He waited till she was on her warpath out of the kitchen before he made his protest.

—It's not right acting like this when I bring one of me friends home.

—Take your tablets, just take your fucking tablets and don't be fucking annoying my arse.

—We'll go for a pizza, Paul.

We had the pizza in the van.

—We'll give Mary time to cool down. Women, hah, you can't live without them and you can't live with them. She'll be grand when we go back.

Just to make sure we bought thirty-six cans of lager in the Westerner where Bumper and the boss man seemed to be best buddies again and the hatchet mark on the counter had been varnished over. Mary accepted Bumper's peace offering without saying thanks and stayed staring at a video that was based on a true story. She talked when she got drunk and slid down from the arm of the chair to sit in Bumper's lap. He patted the tarnished silver stud in her nose.

The sitting-room was all ex-army sleeping bags and blankets draped over the bits of furniture. Bumper said you'd never know who'd pop in but no one did. I realized this was where I wanted to stay the night when the last can was bocked up and thrown into the corner. Bumper got a tremor that made his body seem to change position inside his skin. Mary cradled his head in her lap.

—Are you all right?

—I will be. I'm just thinking of Noelie beyond in Temple-keeran with the worms eating at him.

—Don't think about it, darling.

—Ahhh, Noelie and this man's brother, down in the ground, holy fuck.

Bumper got off his chair and paced the room a couple of times. He seemed a small bit calmer when he sat down.

—We'll kill them, Bumper, don't worry.

It sounded like my voice but it floated away in front of me like an astronaut adrift in deep space. Bumper and Mary clinked empty lager cans together.

—We'll sort them all right, Paul, I have it worked out. There'll be some sorry fuckers in Abbeytown, especially Fuck Doggy Dog Giff.

—And this famous big fella.

—And him too. He's surely getting it.

The shiver and shake left Bumper. He hoisted his wife into his arms and staggered for the door.

—Let yourself out. I'm in the mood for action.

I didn't stir. I only sat there looking at a blank TV screen and wishing I didn't have to leave this house. Mary knocked on the door. The pile of blankets in front of her was bigger than herself and in better shape than the ones already in the room.

—Here you go, throw these over you and sleep on the settee. Action Man sparked out when the head hit the pillow. You'll hardly make it home in the state you're in.

I felt safe for a second before I fell into the dark. We had a purpose now. That purpose was Snoopy Giff. Johnny, all that was going to be done for you.

But I didn't dream of Johnny or of Snoopy Giff in his monkey mask, although I tried to as the lager scorched my mind in and out of sleep and made me uncertain which was the real world and which a dream or whether there were two such categories at all.

Always the same dream. Always. Again. In thirst.

Here he is again. The boy who used to be me tramping along this country road. In that same cheap T-shirt and shorts. The dry, dusty road with the fields of green grass running parallel to it. The heat haze rising up off the road. My parched tongue swelling up and paining my mouth.

Then I find the pump. The old blue one. I pull the handle and the water flows from the pump. Silver water like brand-new coins. Water that sparkles in the sun like it does on telly ads. The most refreshing drink I ever had. Clear country water in my mouth and in my hair and all over my face. It kills my thirst.

Eleven

I'm the Lawnmower

I never could sleep in strange beds. Couches a foot wide are even worse. The blunt bleat of the early-bird train decided me on getting up. The only sound in the house came from a cistern that couldn't make up its mind whether to go for a full gurgle or not. The only sound outside in the Diamond came from a horse kicking her hooves against the tin walls of a fuel shed.

The only car moving in the place at that hour was the one parked opposite the Westerner. A cop car. It followed me for a hundred yards before pulling up ahead of me. The smart-casual detective opened the back door and pointed at the seat. I stopped dead where I was and shook my head. As much to clear it as to say no.

—Come on, Mr Kelly, we want a few words with you in the station.

—What about?

—About what do you think? It's hardly about a fucking dog licence.

—I don't want to talk to you.

—It's your own choice, buddy. We can't make you come in and talk to us but we could come down and visit you at home.

—The kettle is always on the boil. Anyways my home is in London.

—Smart lad. We could turn up on your mammy's door-step with a search warrant and turn the place over twice looking for something we couldn't find. But don't let me pressurize you, Paul.

The pig in the back of the squad hadn't shaved yet. Hairy bacon.

—I'm as fucking tired, to be honest with you. This caper has me fagged out.

A few snatches of singing came from one of the cells. It sounded like Ozzie Small's voice. The gaff reminded me of the King William an hour and a half before opening time. A cold, quiet building waiting impatiently for people to fill it with heat and noise.

—If you could step this way, please, Mr Kelly.

The stubbly guard broke into a spectacular yawn the second after he eked out my name. Surprising just how cold the station was. Water droplets in the air and ridges of damp underneath the peeling wallpaper of the room we entered.

The set-up reminded me of the brewery interview board that allocated the good pubs. Smart-Casual sat behind the table beside two uniforms and a silver-haired man in a long green coat who had his feet planked up on the table and was fucking around at cat's cradles with a lump of string He had very big feet. Even for a cop.

—We'd like if you'd make a statement.

—A statement about what? The plight of the sperm whale?

—For fuck's sake.

The detective's fist was on its way down to pound the table when the man with the silver hair looked over at him. His hand froze in mid-air for a couple of seconds before he laid it down palm first on the table and spread out his fingers. The man with the silver hair went back to cat's cradles.

—We'd like to know what you know about the recent murders in Rathbawn.

—We'd like to know why there's been two murders and a few more attempted murders. You have a bit of cop on, you're a sensible man and we think you might be able to tell us what's going on.

The detective leaned across the table. I suppose he thought he was snarling.

—We want to know why you're hanging around with that scumbag Bumper Reilly. Ye're at something, we know ye are. And we want to know what it is.

—I'm saying nothing. We're not up to anything. I'm just meeting him the odd time for a few oul pints.

The man with the silver hair left a perfect cat's cradle on the table in front of him. He shrugged the green coat off his back and on to the back of his chair.

—Maybe you don't know anything. But we think you know who was behind the killings of your brother Johnny and Noel Reilly. Maybe you do. Maybe you don't. Do you?

I shook my head. Maybe it was the drink from the night before that didn't let me trust my voice. He rubbed one hairy hand against the side of his schnozz.

—If you know you really should tell me. This situation could turn very nasty and a lot more people could be killed if it doesn't stop soon. Savvy?

The English expression made me smile. The detective

leaned across the table and hit me a rap across the mouth. It didn't land that well but the smell of aftershave from his fist and the metallic pong of his signet rings made me gag. My eyes filled up with water so I stared at the floor. When I looked up, the man with the silver hair was telling the detective to take a walk and cool down.

—That's police brutality, that is.

—No, it's not, son. Believe me, it's not. That's just someone being tetchy in the morning. Listen to me, I've got to know as much as I can about this whole caper because I've a feeling it's a different league from what you boys are used of.

He ripped the cat's cradles apart. Something about the register of his voice made me wonder who or what he was and what the crack was with him. His hands were behind his head when he continued.

—We could tell your buddy there, ould Bumper, that you split on him. We could say you put him in the frame for a few robberies and a bit of receiving. Then we could let him roam around on the loose for a bit. He'd have your guts for garters. So I'm saying to you again to tell us what you know. I know you won't believe me but it's in your best interests. And I'm fed up playing good cop.

—I can't tell you anything because I don't know anything about this. I'm only over from beyond a short while. I'm like Manuel, I know nothing.

I felt a bit more confident. I knew the last thing Bumper would do was let me down. I knew he knew the same about me. If the buck was playing his trump card his hand was full of shit.

He looked down at his hands. The two uniforms twitched nervously on the chairs. They didn't look at him. They looked anywhere where they couldn't see him. A tap on the door.

—There's a solicitor outside, he says he's this man's solicitor, said a Ban Garda.

Badger Bonce raised his eyebrows and then stared at me. Very hard like he knew I was starting to get smart with him inside in my head.

—It's John Flynn, sir.

—I don't really need to be around here, boys.

The Indian Elephant, the Silver Fox, the Grey Mule. Whoever. He slipped out the door like the star of the greasy pig competition at Sheepwalk parish sports. The bluebottles shifted position on their chairs like a ten-ton lead weight had been removed from their shoulders. I suppose ten tons of feathers would have been as heavy. But lead sounds more painful. Although feathers would have made them sneeze and it looked like they would have been afraid to do even that in front of the string specialist, whoever he was.

I hadn't seen John Flynn since he advised me that assuring Judge Conlon of my emigratory intentions was the best hope of avoiding a stint in a bunk with a Dublin joyrider underneath me. He'd jacked all that shit in now. His last eight years were a carnival of pieces of wood in loaves of bread, nails in Danish pastries, shop signs that flew back and hit people in the face when the wind got up and unsafe roadworks that made motorbikes crash. He lived on the Dublin Road now. Between the Church of Ireland hall and Senator Mullaney's house. He was mouthing off about the rights of the individual, civil liberties and the going rate for post-traumatic stress disorder when the two cops got me to the front door of the barracks.

—I'm very worried that my client was brought here against his will.

—He wasn't, Mr Flynn. And he never said he was your client.

—That remains to be seen.

Flynn redid the knot on his tie when he saw the Ban Garda.

—I hope you haven't made a statement.

I wondered if I owed him money for this. And what the fuck was going on here. And was the whole place gone fucking mad. By the time Flynn finished bollocking any convenient cops they were apologizing to me. I let a shout at the pair from the quiz session as we walked out.

—It's a pity there isn't a third one of ye or I'd huff and I'd puff and I'd blow yere house down.

A job lot from the EC disdain surplus coloured Flynn's voice.

—You're not that clever, you know. Don't ever let yourself be brought in there again without a solicitor.

He handed me his card before he got into his BMW. I knocked on the window as he turned the key in the ignition.

—I'm sorry, Mr Kelly. I can't give you a lift. I'm not a taxi service, you know.

—No. It's not that. How did you know where I was?

—Your friend, the famous Mr Reilly, engaged me to look after your interests. You might say I owe him one.

—How did he know where I was?

—He knew. He knows what's going on.

—Everyone in this town knows everything that's going on.

—Except you, Mr Kelly.

Interrogation leaves you stressed out. Stressed out enough to need a pint. I bought a *Star* and sat under the monument looking at the racecards. Twenty minutes of a wait before the sound of the bolt being drawn back. I knew after the first pint that I needed one more. Enough to set me daydreaming. Because Lydia's face was threatening to wash up on shore again.

—And a large brandy with that, Joe.

Bumper poured the brandy into the sink when he arrived. He said he'd replace it when the night's work was finished.

—We're going to see Snoopy Giff.

But we didn't drive out the road to Abbeytown when we left Donoghue's. We drove past the Diamond and turned up a laneway pitted with spiderwebs of potholes that twice nearly turned the car over. Bumper jumped over a log barrier and into a rutted field when we stopped. I followed him across the field.

—No more what's up doc for bucky here.

A small dirty-grey rabbit in a wire snare. A thin smear of blood across his nose and mouth. His leg twisted underneath him at a wishbone angle. I turned my back but I still heard the tearing sound. Bumper admired his hands and threw Bugs into the plastic bag we used to carry the drink from the Westerner the night before.

He left the engine running when he jumped out of the car outside his house and ran around to the fuel shed. A thick white fertilizer bag was in his hands when he came back. Flies buzzed around the mouth of the bag. Bloated blue flies whose song sounded deliberately aggressive. A strange lion's-cage smell came from the bag. I asked Bumper what was in it. All he did was smile and put a finger up to his lips. The flies kept buzzing. Even when the bag was thrown into the boot where the spare tyre should have been. They hung around outside the boot. Jilted. It was a beautiful evening. We hit for Abbeytown and Snoopy Giff.

The Abbey Bar was quiet. A couple of youngsters raced ponies in the street outside. A light breeze took the heat of my face and made it feel white instead of red.

I made to sit down at the first stool we came to. Bumper kept walking. I followed him again. He strolled into the lounge where music played and the pint was five pence dearer. I wondered why Bumper hadn't said anything about weapons. I wondered again about the contents of the white fertilizer bag.

There was only one customer in this part of the Abbey Bar and I knew who he was before we got near him. The barman was leaning over the counter and listening with attention so undivided it had to be put on. Myself and Bumper walked in step now. Side by side. Mick Flavin sang on the jukebox about love and the stars.

The shamrock shaved into the back of Snoopy's head bobbed up and down in a punchy way as he talked. We came up behind him at the bar. I thought of how he must have searched the Dandy Diner that night for the back of Beetlejuice's head. Another night he had searched for the back of Johnny's head. Bumper raised his hand as he passed behind him. Snoopy turned around and I realized he didn't know who Bumper was. Bumper snapped his hand into a salute to the barman.

—Could we have a couple of pints there, head?

The tattoos were the first thing you noticed. From a distance each of his arms looked covered with a single long blue birthmark. But they were his tattoos. From Loughan. How much glass? How much blood?

They were mainly of girls' faces. Girls with big, round, blue eyes whose hair was long and stringy and parted in the middle. Snakes, scorpions and Thin Lizzy's Black Rose there as well. A cartoon cat stood on his hind legs above each elbow, wearing a top hat and carrying a cane. The barman served us while making sure to keep looking at Snoopy and faking interest.

—So I says, motherfucker, you and your homies come into my hood again and you're fucking dead meat, boy. Your ass is grass and I'm the lawnmower. Like fuck you, maaan.

The same bad American accent. The voice that shouted in the Dandy Diner. Bumper saw the recognition in my eyes.

He was happy Robbie Lawrence had been scared enough to tell him the truth.

Bumper raised his hand behind Snoopy's head. I clenched my fists. Ready for the action. Bumper plunged his arm forward and took our drinks from the barman. He signalled to me to do nothing. Yet. We sat a few feet away from our man and tried not to make anything too obvious.

Some of our man's mates came into the music lounge and sat down silently while he talked at them. They drifted away after a bit. But Snoopy's voice kept going. Like an unattended burglar alarm in the night. Every time he came to the main point of the joke or story he brought his arm forward and engraved the air with a sign. His two extreme fingers pointed outwards and his thumb bent slightly.

—Snoop Doggy Dog, boys, Snoop Doggy Dog.

The same Utah Jazz cap on his head. Turned to the side. A jacket with LA Raiders in relief letters across the back. And those wide trousers with the black and white striped cloth at the knees. His Troop hi-tops would have made even Kaya's feet look size fourteen.

Me and Bumper didn't talk. Not even to each other. We just watched. And drank. Very slowly. Snoopy drank enough to soon leave only coppers in the big pockets of those trousers. The barman gave him two pints on the house. I think he might have hesitated for a moment when he got asked for a third. Snoopy was sure he did which was why he leaned in over the counter and got a grip of his neck. The barman tried to apologize but there was so much of his windpipe in Snoopy's fist he couldn't dredge up anything intelligible. Snoopy wasn't in the humour for listening anyways. He put the sign in the air again.

—Can you kick it G? Can you kick it?

A few of the couples who'd just come in to the music lounge went doorwards. Snoopy cleared his throat greenly and started chanting

She want the baddest motherfucker
And who's that, sucker?
Baddest fucker in the whole damn hood
Mess with me it won't do you no good
What do they call me?

He slackened his grip on the barman's neck and relapsed into an Abbeytown accent.

—What do they call me Peter?

—Snoop Doggy Dog.

—Yeah. Snoop Doggy Dog, you dig?

Snoopy turned around and looked Bumper straight in the eye. Bumper looked straight back.

—Not since I left the County Council road gang.

They stared each other down in silence for a few seconds and turned their eyes away at the same moment.

Snoopy Giff didn't have to buy any more drinks before closing time. People in the bar made their bodies compact and pulled their shoulders in when he walked past them. We were out the front door ten seconds after him. He walked up the hill towards the shopping centre carpark. We kept a hundred yards behind him. He was chanting away to himself so he probably couldn't hear us. He never looked behind. The hi-tops made no sound on the ground. Snoopy Giff floated noiselessly along in front of us like the ghost he was soon going to be.

We were just fifty yards behind him when he started fumbling for his car keys. The carpark was almost empty. It all seemed too easy. He was on his own in the dark section with not a soul in sight. But Bumper walked past Snoopy's car. And I followed him.

We sat into Bumper's car. Bumper looked ultra-relaxed. Like a Radox bath on legs. I shook and waited for the next move. I was shitting it now. I just kept telling myself this had to be done.

Snoopy's car stereo lacerated the silence. His car bounced up and down like a low rider. We followed him out of the carpark. Bumper hummed snatches of ballads and giggled for no reason I could see. Snoopy turned into an estate behind an old people's home with small vandalized trees in front of it. We waited for him to park before we stopped. A hundred yards. The sound system stayed booming.

A couple of lights came on in the estate. Some curtains flicked back. The lights went off again pronto and the curtains swayed back logically to stand between the houses and the street. Someone turned an upstairs light on in the little house Snoopy had parked outside. The door opened a few seconds later. A reluctant stream of light dribbled down the path. Snoopy killed the booming system and stepped out of the car.

A skinny woman in floral pyjamas advanced halfway down the path to meet him. They embraced in a hurry. Her feet were bare. Her hands sat on his shoulders and back like they belonged to a climber seeking a hold on a treacherous rock face. I recognized her when she stepped back. Bubblicious Doherty.

Bumper lit two fags from the car lighter and handed me one. His voice was thoughtful. You could have mistaken it for gentle if the glowing tip of the fag hadn't lit up his face.

—Sit tight, Paul, he'll hardly be more than half an hour.

—What's in the white bag in the boot?

—You'll see soon. I wonder does he do the job Snoopy Dog Doggy-style.

It was an hour before Snoopy came out of the house. Bubblicious snogged him on the doorstep for a full five minutes. I wondered if Johnny's last hours alive had been like this. Maybe with Theresa Lawrence. The door closed. The outside light flickered and died. Snoopy staggered down the path and sang to himself.

He had that look of the other world about him. The look that comes after love and sex and usually stays hidden behind sleeping eyelids. Bumper's right leg started shaking and produced a staccato rattle from the floor of the car. I unlocked my door. I felt a pang of guilt about killing a man just after he left his girlfriend. Killing him when he was maybe at his best. I was almost out of my seat when Bumper threw me back into it and locked my door again.

—Didn't I tell you to hold fucking tight.

Snoopy half strolled and half danced into his Mazda 323. He set his system at maximum bass for Ice Cube and drove off. And all Bumper did was put his hand up to his mouth to stifle a yawn. He didn't move until the sound of the music had left the night and the thump of the bass stopped shaking the pits of our stomachs.

No lights were on in the estate now. None got switched on when Bumper jumped out of the car and opened the boot. He brought a bag into the car. Not the white bag. The bag with the rabbit in it. Bugs was starting to pong fairly fucking choice. Bumper told me to switch on the inside light. He sat in the back seat and pulled a butcher's knife off the back window. One quick arm movement was enough to cut the head off the rabbit and send red swirling among the blue and green patterns of the rug covering the back seat.

—Shall I carve? said Bumper in a bad attempt at a Lord Snooty accent.

I laughed despite myself. And despite the fact my stomach seemed to be trying to escape through the floor via my feet. The smell of the rabbit jammed right inside the top of my nose the way crusts of dried blood do after a nosebleed. I wanted to get out of the car. But I stayed and watched Bumper. Carving. One leg off. Then another. Another. Another. I thought of the front legs as the rabbit's arms. It took a good while for Bumper to finish. All the lights in the houses stayed off except for occasional one- and five-minute illuminations of late jaunts to the jacks.

After he slit open the stomach, Bumper carefully removed the entrails and sprinkled them along the length of the body. This time I turned away and switched on *The Leuuve Zone*. But I didn't know the song. I turned round again. Bumper was wrapping pieces of the rabbit up in the pages of the *Sun* we'd taken from outside McDonnell's the morning after our first tour of the countryside.

Bumper was the boss. He knew what he was at.

—Remind me to throw that fucking rug away when we're out the road.

The smell wouldn't let either of us forget.

—Now watch this.

Bumper carried the newspaper parcel carefully as he walked towards Bubblicious's house. The parcel rested on the front wall while he vaulted the gate with one hand.

Not a sound abroad in the night. Bumper signalled to me to drive the car up. It was that quiet the sound of the engine seemed to ring around the country. I suddenly realized what we were going at. What Bumper was going at. I'm not backing off from blame. It's just I never had a clue of half of what he planned. It mightn't have made any difference. Bumper was the pro. He would make sense of it for me.

He legged it out to the car when I arrived. The upstairs lights had come on in the house. In two different rooms. Bumper panted. His words came out between breaths.

—Stall the digger here for a minute. Hoot the horn a couple of times. She'll get a quare fright when she comes out the door.

The horn sounded twice. Then again. The hall light came on. I heard a child bawling its head off as the front door opened. Bubblicious's face peeped out.

—Hoot the horn again.

Bumper thumped me on the arm. I sounded the horn

again. Bubblicious stepped forward. She looked at the car. Then she looked down. I followed her gaze.

A scream burst out of somewhere deep where there were no controls. Another scream followed it up. More screams. The sound of the child crying in the house was louder now. Bubblicious stumbled around the path for a few seconds. Lashing out at invisible enemies. She bent over and screamed in the dry voice of babies afflicted with breathing ailments that make them go rapidly red in the face. Lights flicked on in some of the other houses. But no one came out. Someone made it as far as their front door, brushed their hand against the lock and then thought better of it.

—Aaaaaaaaaaaah aaaaaaaaah aaaaaaaahahahahahahaahhh-haaa.

Bubblicious looked out at the car and glanced down the street as if there was somewhere she could run to. Her dressing-gown had come undone. Her stomach showed a pregnant curve. Bumper rocked with a silent laughter that made the passenger seat move backwards and forwards. The little rubbery creaks annoyed me. Bubblicious backed towards the door and looked down in horror again as she walked through the mess of rabbit remains. This scream would have served as a definition of hysterical for the alien who landed in your back garden and asked for one.

She left the door open as she scrambled up the stairs. I could see into the hall. A fakey gold hairbrush hung beside a matching wall mirror. Her tiny white feet. Size threes? Her tiny white feet scuttled towards the door. She closed it. We heard her check twice to make sure it was locked. Her bare feet had scattered the rabbit all over the garden path. I tried to pick out some pattern but there wasn't one.

A feeling was in the car along with us when we parked outside the Marian Grotto. A strong, sour feeling. Bumper opened two bottles of Harp with his teeth. I wanted to go home. Any home. The right thing to do at this moment would be to pick Kaya up, hug her and swing her around in the air. We didn't listen to the radio.

The smell of the dead animal was on Bumper's hands. It took over the whole car. All the air being hugged by this red-raw stink that made me think of the way a Portugese graveyard up in the mountains had smelled when me and Lydia passed it on a day of almost visible heat. I wished it was time for the birds to start the dawn chorus and let us know the worst of the night was over.

—Drive back.

—What?

—Drive back. To yer one's house. The crack isn't over yet.

The dark in the estate was broken now. By one light in the bedroom window of Bubblicious's house. And another light left on in her hall. The idea maybe being to make intruders think she was up and keep them away from the house. She hadn't copped that these intruders wanted her to be up.

Maybe she was in the hall. Sitting at a table. Drinking coffee because the urge for sleep had been frightened out of her. Counting out the minutes until it was morning enough for her to gather up the kids and make a run for it somewhere, though it didn't exactly seem like there was any place to head towards. She could be sat in front of the goldy mirror. Brushing the same strands of hair so she had something to do with her shaking hands.

Or maybe she was sleeping sound on her back like a queen. This sort of crack might happen to her the whole time. She might keep Snoopy's guns for him. Bumper fossicked around in the boot. She probably drove Snoopy around on his jobs. All fair in the revenge game. But she didn't have a car.

Bumper knocked on my door. I rolled down the window. He held something in his right hand. Behind his back.

—Moo, said Bumper.

The fright jumped me backwards and across the car. Something seemed to twist and give in my back. A rapid stream of farts filled the car with the smell of a manky pub jacks.

—Moo. Alas, poor Daisy, I knew her well.

The cow had a fairly happy expression. As much as you can judge these things from the look of a severed head. Maybe there's a bovine equivalent to these European euthanasias where you have a couple of glasses of wine with a civilized blondy chap named Johann before he does the jab.

Where did Bumper get the head from? Factories kill cows the whole time and throw away the heads. So they had to be easy enough got only I couldn't get rid of the picture of him stalking across the fields of Sheepwalk with a scythe under his arm.

A couple of white maggots had burrowed into a little trench under the eyes. The smell of blood amazed me. That and the size of the ears. And the whiskers under the chin.

—Moo, said Bumper again.

He leaned against the car so amusement at his own wit wouldn't knock him over.

—I was going skinning it and just leaving the skull but I think she looks better this way. What do you reckon?

I had the keys in the ignition before the thought that this had something to do with Johnny, my dead brother that I loved, kept me where I was. I watched Bumper jam the head on to one side of the gate and remembered that this was for better or for worse. The sight of the maggots made my skin itch. A cold sweat bonded my clothes to me. A taste like week-old black coffee had come in my mouth. It stopped me talking to Bumper when he got back into the car. Panic.

—Hit the horn a clatter there, good boy.

I did what I was told. No sign of life in the house. Bumper went in and clattered the front door a few times. No reply. No nothing. He thumped his head off the dashboard and hit the radio a slap. Something broke and rattled loose.

—Fuck it, I don't even want her to come to the door. All I want the fucking bitch to do is look out, can she not even do that much for me?

We waited. We made more noise. The house stayed quiet. It began to get light outside. I thought she must have scarpered just after we left the first time and left the lights on to fool us. Cheat. Then I noticed a shadow sit up and move behind the curtains of the upstairs room with the light on. It was a few seconds before I told Bumper.

—I'll tell you what I'll do. I'll toss a bit of a stone against that window. She might think it's someone she knows like Giff or someone.

He scratched around on the footpath for a bit before jumping over a wall three doors down and coming back with a prime exhibit from someone's rock garden. The trajectory of his throw was a long ways too flat. The rock shattered the glass. Bubblicious forgot everything else and looked out. The Africa-shaped hole in the window framed her face perfectly. She looked like she'd pulled a muscle in her mind. We'd reminded her of what her life was.

That was why both her hands were planted in her hair and she was gulping to get in what now seemed like much thinner air. Bumper had known all this would happen. He knew people. But he needed to see her. To see her seeing the head. He had no imagination. He was a happy man on the journey home.

—Perfect, Paul, fucking perfect.

—Hah?

—We'll make Snoopy Giff suffer, you see. He'll find out how much of a man he is for his family.

—When are we going to do Giff?

—Take your time, there's any amount of it.

—It's Giff who killed Johnny and Noelie. Giff and this famous big man.

—Oh, we'll sort Giff all right. Only there's a few ways to go about it before he buys the farm.

—There's more than one way to skin a cat.

—There is aye only, fuck it, I never checked to see if yer one had a cat.

I listened to myself laughing and maybe for a second I wondered how we could do this to a pregnant woman who we didn't even know. Then I thought of how much had happened to the most perfect woman who ever lived and how it made this seem like nothing. And I didn't worry any more. That made this seem like nothing.

Liverpool were playing on the first worst day of my life. I remember that because the game was exciting enough for me to leave the bar so I could watch it in peace upstairs. I went for a slash in the break before the experts came on to tell me what I had been looking at.

The jacks door was open. Lydia sat propped up against the toilet. I knew what I was looking at even before I picked the needle up off the red carpet she spent so much time agonizing over. A year earlier.

I knew too she'd made a fuck out of her first attempts at the injection. A purple stain where a vein gave up the ghost. It wasn't the only mark on her arms. A smell of shit and puke overpowered Beautiful by Estée Lauder. But it didn't eliminate it. Lydia was looking at me and she wasn't. Drool flowed down the centre of her chin. I wiped it away carefully with a piece of toilet paper and dragged her into the sitting-room. She felt like the air had been let out of her. I put her lying on the couch. For a split second I thought of watching the action replay to see who got the goal. I switched the telly off. Another excuse to curse myself in the morning. Ian Rush.

I belled an ambulance. And a cab as well in case the ambulance service lived up to the horror tales of the time. Vinnie cleared the pub. As if he'd expected this. I rode in the ambulance with Lydia. A tall glass in my hand. Joan gave it to me as we waited. Three brandies in the glass. Eejit. No. Idiot. I had the accent nearly lost by then. She'd worked in pubs all her life and she still didn't cop that drink doesn't get rid of misery. It just moves it into a different time zone. Sometimes.

Lydia's eyes fluttered like a butterfly trapped behind glass as the traffic cleared out of the way. I didn't want them to shut. It was a short run to the hospital. One of the porters, a red-haired sketch from Donegal who drank in the King William, saluted me cheerfully as I walked in behind the trolley.

What was I like?

When we pushed through the first set of clinging Perspex doors Lydia's eyes opened wide and rolled up wildly like they were going to go out the back of her head. Then they closed. I wanted them to close now. The ambulance men talked to her. All the way down through the hospital to Accident and Emergency.

They told her she was a great girl. To hold on. She'd be all right. She was a great girl.

Maybe they said this to everyone. But I thought they could see there was something special about Lydia. She didn't belong on this trolley with one of her punctured arms hanging out over the side. Her face was so white her hair looked impossibly black. White foam covered her lips.

—You may kiss the bride.

A doc asked me if I knew my wife had a heroin problem. I

said I didn't. I hadn't. He told me there were rehabilitation programmes which offered addicts a good chance of recovery. Especially in the early stages of addiction.

I was halfway up the stairs of the pub the next morning when I remembered I'd forgotten to ask anyone to look after Kaya. Vinnie was beside the cot. Half-asleep with his big fist around a bottle and a rattle at his feet. I woke him up. So I could cry into his shoulder. He told me there were things I could take. But all I wanted to do was cry on him. The rules had been changed and nobody had told me. Or they had always been different to what I thought.

It was almost the same world the next morning. The women in the kitchen still clanked bits of cutlery together and rattled dishes. I was in hell. Vinnie was chalking up the lunch menu on the board outside. The octogenarian who claimed to be Grand Master of the Freemasons rolled up his right trouser leg and hopped around the public bar. Small flecks of blood hung around the rim of the toilet bowl. Lydia was in a comfortable condition. With an intravenous drip hanging out of her.

I brought a mixed bouquet the first day I visited her. She burrowed her head into the pillow and refused to talk to me. On the second day she said she was sorry and I bent to kiss her chapped lips. I brought her twelve red roses and they stood proud in water when I left. They were gone the next day. The ward sister didn't answer me when I asked what happened to them. But she was polite about it.

When Lydia came home I brought her down the Greek and ordered champagne which I spluttered out on to the tablecloth when she told me a couple of jokes she heard in hospital. I was hopeful for maybe two days. No. Wrong. Wrong wrong wrong. I was hopeful for ever. But I believed for maybe two days. Fact.

It could have been different if she'd been the one who found the young couple from Belfast that time in the Flock of Swans. You wonder. Of course you wonder about all sorts. But still. The pair of them dead in the ladies'. And their little three-year-old son sitting quietly in the lounge with a brightly coloured lollipop stuck in his gob. The cop looked in pain when he took my statement.

—Heroin. I suppose it's just as well this little blighter was here. If he'd been at home he would probably have starved to death before we found out where these two lived.

I'd never thought of anything being that powerful. It frightened me. The calm and silence of the kid when the cop brought him away made me wonder what he was used to.

I used ask Lydia why she took the stuff. And didn't she know I loved her. If she'd even given me a bad reason it might have been easier, but all she did was look at the ground and sniff through a nose that looked raw round the edges.

—I don't know. I'll stop, I'll stop, I'm telling you I'll stop, won't you believe me?

So when does a person become so different that they're not the same person? At all. How far can they go before they've changed enough for you to stop loving them?

Can you stop? At all.

After the woman I still loved flogged our jointly bought CD player, our telly and video and most of Kaya's toys I locked up everything valuable. She couldn't work in the bar because she couldn't be let near the till. The customers got used to her occasional staggers around the public bar without her make-up. Vinnie would hustle her gently back up the stairs.

I popped pills to stay awake at night so I could stop her sneaking out and doing more damage to herself. Some nights she'd wake up and scream and claw at visions on the wall. It might have been most nights. I'm too tired to remember.

So what can anyone do when they find the perfect half to complete the circle and one night you try to stop them banging their head off the wall and you find your hands are all slippy with their blood?

I booked her into the expensive rehab programmes. But she just walked out the other side of them.

What was she thinking as she flapped through the Brixton streets in a nightshirt and slippers? How much did she remember of what her life was?

There are some things in what's left of people's lives that you can't imagine. What was it like for her? That is what I can't know.

I walked up from Dhillon's corner shop one day with a bag of loaves under my oxter. Lydia passed me on the other side of the road. With Dublin Sean. Arm in arm. Now everyone was able to tell me he was one of the biggest pushers on the fucking manor. People always want to tell you things. As if you're fucking interested. As if it does you any good to know things. You're better off in the dark. It's the only place to be. It's yer only man, the oul dark.

Someone had to tell me she'd started hanging round the Brown Cow. The villains' pub. A man shot his best friend there because the geezer stood on his dog's tail. On hot summer days they put chairs on the footpath outside and people crossed over to the other side of the street.

In the dark. I sat in our car in the dark one night outside the Brown Cow. The car Lydia would have sold if the guy on the Walworth Road hadn't got suspicious and rung me at the pub.

It was two o'clock when she came out. Herself and a couple of women rigged out in short, tattered denim minis and mile-high stilettos. Surrounded by a gang of men in old suit jackets with T-shirts underneath them. Lydia's laugh split the night air. Into little splinters of heartbreak. It was high and nervy but it was still her laugh. It made me close my eyes and give up. I leaned against the steering wheel and the horn sounded. Nobody noticed.

Lydia was draped round this villain from Kennington whose hair was a mix of the blondy dye he used to mask his age and the rampant grey that kept showing it. Her hands crawled under his T-shirt. He shook her off and put one unsteady hand against the door of the pub as he pissed against it. He nearly fell before he clasped one hand hard against her arse and staggered down the street. Her leg flinched. Sean came out of the pub in a white suit and called Lydia.

—Lydia. Fuck you, Lydia.

Her name turned to shite in his mouth. She tottered back towards him. Moving inexpertly on the stilettos. Sean held out his hand. Lydia reached into her cleavage and handed him some money. She threw her hands out awkwardly and kissed him. The pair of them held that pose for a few seconds in the reflected light from inside the Brown Cow. He slapped her face hard when she broke away and skidded desperately down the street after her amigos. I couldn't start the car. I couldn't do anything except wait for the light to scare me back to the King William.

—Lydia. Fuck you, Lydia.

—You may kiss the bride.

Most of my minutes that time were spent thinking about killing Sean. I wondered about guns and knives and every other kind of yoke like I was trying to guess the murder weapon in Cluedo. But I knew it was all daft. It wasn't something I could do. It wasn't in me. Not back then.

A heroin addict. That was what they would say Kaya's mother had been. An explanation for the ruins of her life. I couldn't hack that.

I wanted Kaya to be middle-class. To own her own home, be fairly posh and have a job it takes you at least half an hour to do yourself up for in the morning. That was what kept me going.

I reckoned I'd given her a good start. I ran my own

business. Boys and girls from Chichester and Hemel Hemp-
stead and Burnham-on-Crouch worked for me. They had
nice accents and for one reason or another they worked in
my pub now. For me. People who wrote books and made
sculptures that looked like nothing drank in the lounge and
played on the cricket team. I got to wear a suit and eat steak
in restaurants where you could surprise people and make
them smile by leaving a big tip. Kaya went to pre-school.

Which was why I didn't want to see her. What I was
pissing away wasn't what was left of my life. It was what was
left of my dreams. Dreams of Kaya heading intelligently off
to college with a fancy folder full of arcane learning under
one arm and the *New Musical Express* under the other. And I
couldn't stick seeing Kaya realizing what was happening. She
would too realize. Even though she was four. Because she
was intelligent. Kerrie said she was. Without prompting
from me.

Twelve

A Person Out of Water

Bumper wouldn't tell me why we came back to Abbeytown the next day. He did open the boot to show there were no dead beasts in it this time.

The Market Bar was beside the cattle mart. They were lucky that way in Abbeytown. The pub was allowed open at five in the morning. For the farmers. No waiting for the healer in Abbeytown. Whenever you walked into the pub there was an ancient bogman at one end of the bar who seemed just about to fall down and another at the other end eating the pattern off a plate of steak and onions. Abbeytown was that sort of a make of a kind of a place.

We were playing darts against two men in dirty tweed jackets. We stuck down a few pound stake and lost both games. I had an uneasy feeling Bumper meant us to lose. He only took eleven darts to get down to sixteen when he played a singles match against the man whose wispy tash was chewed on both sides. Then he missed the double that would have won him the game. Ten times. It was an awful obvious caper. He was letting me know the fix was in. Myself and the other man talked about England as Bumper unerringly directed his shots to various points six inches from the correct spot.

—What part were you in?

—South London. Brixton.

—Full of blacks.

—Yeah.

—You'd want to paint yourself with boot polish before you'd go out.

—Yeah. I suppose so all right.

—When I went over there in the Fifties, there wasn't a darkie in the place. It was a great spot then. Then they landed. They ruined a sight of places. East London, south London, good addresses, wrecked them all so no one else would live there.

—Begod.

—Of course, you can't say nigger now. Or coon. Because of the liberals. You have to call them men of colour or something like that.

—It's some country.

—Of course, the Brits aren't great themselves. They all have it in for Paddy. There's a lot of what do you call it, racialism, about the place.

Bumper arrived with a tray of pints. He'd settled the bet in jar. The four of us sat back in our chairs. It went quiet for a second.

—Brendan Murtagh.

Bumper put his hand out in a friendly fashion to the man who'd been beyond in England.

—Joseph O'Dowd.

I spoke quickly enough to fool anyone who'd believe Bumper was a bad enough darts player to miss ten doubles in a row.

—Terry Giff.

The man who'd been beyond in England.

—Donie Giff.

The man with the chewed black tash.

I followed Bumper to the jacks when he went. Terry Giff was left with the punchline of a joke dangling in the air. Bumper tried to coax some sort of discharge from the soap dispenser on the wall. Beside the dispenser was a machine full of Red Dragon Pheromone Capsules which contained the irresistible essence of sexual attraction. It must have been true. The *Sunday Express* said so. On no account were you to drink the contents.

—What's going on here then?

—What do you mean?

—Who are the two boys?

—Terry Giff is Snoopy's oul fella and Donie Giff is his uncle.

—Fuck's sake. What are we going doing next?

—Will you ever stop asking me stupid questions?

—What are we going doing next isn't a stupid question.

—It is. It's the stupidest question. How can I know what we're going doing next? I can only know what we're doing now. Anyways, you've probably made a balls of it. It looks shocking suspicious the pair of us going to the jacks at the same time.

Bumper was right. The Giffs were cagier when we came back. We played a few hands of poker. There was less chat and Terry kept complaining he was getting a gammy share. They gulped their whiskies now like they wanted to keep their mouths busy so words weren't expected to come out. The lights in the pub flicked on and off twice.

—Mini power cut. Straight flush.

—No. They do that to show the pub is closing. Royal flush.

—Twenty-one. Pontoon, said Terry Giff.

I think he was serious. I was going to say:

—Rummy.

But I was put off by the fact that canasta means something in Irish and I couldn't think of what it fucking was. No way. I couldn't. Korsakoff's psychosis strikes again. I couldn't. Korsakoff's psychosis strikes again. Whist is the Irish for keep quiet.

—Meself and Joseph are going down to a drinking party by the canal. Do ye want to come?

Bumper made a big deal out of buying a box of cans and plonking it down on the table. The Giffs hummed and hawed and looked up at the rain pissing down and speckling the skylight. Bumper looked up as well. In his head he was climbing across a roof with a cash till under his arm.

—We'll give it a miss, lads. But thanks all the same.

Donie's voice was the friendliest it had been since we came back from the jacks. He leaned against the armrest. Terry grinned sideways at us. They were both seriously out of the game.

The raindrops played taps on the plastic cover of our Foster's box as we zigzagged back to the car.

—Fuck that gobshite Michael Fish. Can he get nothing right, Paul?

—He's like a person out of water.

Bumper giggled. I laughed. He giggled again. That set us off. We had to leave the cans down on the footpath. I had to lean over the bonnet with my shirtsleeves in a pool of rain collected in a fist-sized dunge. The joke or something else was that funny.

—A person out of water. Fuck's sake.

We heard Terry and Donie Giff before we saw them.

—Dublin scum, Dublin cunts, Dublin shit.

—Dublin bastards, you dirty Dublin bastards, mothers five for a pound.

I knew what we were going to do. Or what we thought we might do. Bumper was right. You can't know what you are going to do. But he always seemed to have a fair clue. If he'd bet with Pearce and Prunty on the outcome of the night he would have collected.

The rain got heavier. The boyos had tried to pull their jackets up over their heads for shelter. What they'd succeeded in doing was pulling their shirts out of their trouser waistbands so the rain and wind now beat against their beer bellies and made whatever discomfort loomed through the drink murk even worse.

—Do ye want a lift out home, boys?

They ran in relief to the car and smiled triumphantly when they saw that by complete coincidence it was their two friendly new chums from the Market Bar going out the road the same time as them. It's a funny old world. But you wouldn't want to sit through its stand-up routine.

Bumper got into the back seat and let Donie into the front. He explained this was because he had to get out first. They nodded agreement because it was really throwing it down now and they were drunk and Bumper's statement had the cut of sense about it. They said they lived in Durack Row. When we got to Durack Row Bumper told me to keep driving out the road. Terry didn't notice. Donie twigged sharp.

—Sorry, mate, that's Durack Row in there. You're gone past it.

—Aren't we all?

Bumper sounded cheerful. Terry chuckled.

—It's OK, we can get out up here at this bush. It's the bush stop.

—Good man, Terry, if wit was shit you'd be constipated, said Bumper.

A can cracked open in the dark. Bumper fumbled casually on the back window ledge for something.

—Give us a light there, Paul.

The lights of Durack Row ran away from us. We rounded a bend. The Giff boys had no sight of home now.

—Come on now, lads, ye'll have a few cans out by the canal with us. We'll be lonely if we have no one to drink with, it's nice to have company on a night like this.

The wipers didn't get rid of the rain quick enough. Thick slicks of rain started to clog up the glass. The Giffs were gone a bit uneasy but they still thought all we were was daft and drunk. Their breathing came quicker all the same. Donie's was close to my ear because he was leaning across and trying to get a clear view. He got on my wick.

—Keep driving, Paul, said Bumper.

Past the Canal Amenity Area. Two picnic tables, one swing and a couple of hundred johnnies lying in the grass like the Caucasian cousins of the common slug. Three miles out of town now.

A piece of rubber from the wipers came unstuck and slowed down the action of the left blade. The road was dark. I could see hardly anything. Maybe that was why I did what I did when Donie started screaming.

—Let us out, let us out, ye cunts ye.

He grabbed the steering wheel. He surprised me. And all he did was spin the wheel round in a circle and send the car all the way across to the other side of the road. No car came in the other direction. If one had we would have been killed stone-dead.

I took the fag lighter out from the dash and planted the orange tip down on Donie's hand. I left it there a good while. It slipped as the soft skin gave way and a mark burned into the hand. He let out a yowl and then put his head between his knees. Blubbering and crying. I was embarrassed. So I looked into the back. Bumper was holding a knife to Terry's throat. There was a great shine off the blade.

I wondered if there was something wrong with the engine before I copped the foul smell was coming from Donie's hand. Bumper piped up from behind.

—Ye didn't say ye had a snack box with ye. That smells finger-lickin' good, boys.

A large sign pointed to Abbeytown Cemetery. Bumper told me to turn down by it. Terry tried to make a move in the back. Bumper sounded calm and bored.

—I'd say that lighter would do some job on a man's eye.

The overgrown grass and bushes on either side of the laneway penned us into a sort of Cresta Run with potholes. Abbeytown Cemetery looked way better kept than Templekeeran. Bumper kicked Terry out of the car. I heard the splash as he landed in a pool of water. The rain slanted across in diagonal sheets that looked like a solid wall when Bumper switched the torch on. I pulled Donie out of the front of the car by the hair. There was no need for it. He would have got out himself.

We sent Donie and Terry through a gap in the wall before us. They could have bolted. Neither tried. They stumbled and slithered in the mud as we walked through the graveyard. A squelchy, farty noise told me someone's shoes had filled up with water. The thought that mud had probably caked on the bottom of my jeans annoyed me. I laced Donie on the back of the head. My knuckles hurt.

The place smelt of leaves. Damp fallen leaves piled up and rotting to black. All the air had damp in it. We walked along a narrow gravel path. Between two long headstone avenues. My foot hit something hard on the ground. I heard a sharp crack. I looked down and saw a container of imitation flowers with a diagonal scar running from right to left through the plastic. Jitters all of a sudden even though I don't believe in good or bad luck. Donie slowed down to hardly-moving-at-all speed. He shivered like a current was being run through his back. His hands were up on top of his head though he hadn't been asked to do anything like that.

The torch illuminated a small circle in front of Bumper. A high side wall barred our way and brought us to a standstill beside each other. I knew Bumper hadn't decided where we were going next. Donie Giff dropped stagily. The sound of the gravel ripping one trouser leg came first. Followed by the sound of Donie babbling.

—Where's the drink? Where's the drink? Lads, come on, where's this party ye were bringing us to?

Edgings of hope seeped slowly out of his voice after the first few words. Bumper kicked him hard into the chest. I thought I heard something break but I couldn't be sure because the wind was swirling round and drowning out a lot of the noises.

I stood back and watched Bumper batter them. First Donie. Then Terry. He hammered Donie across the path with his fists until he fell over the iron border of a plot whose white chippings glittered in the torchlight. Bumper tumbled over the iron as well but didn't stop hitting.

He propped Donie up against a headstone and went through his jacket and trousers before filching a wallet, some notes and a few coins which sent strange little lines of light shooting off the stone walls.

The only sounds were Bumper's breaths. And little whimpers out of the Giffs. Terry could still have made a run for it. I would have let him go. But he just stood there stupidly by the wall until Bumper came over and slammed him into it. Bumper dug hard into him with his boots like he was opening a roll of carpet. He went through Terry's pockets and took out another wallet and a rake of plastic cards which must have been useless because he tried to break them. They bent like soft toffee and he fucked them into the long grass by the wall. I landed a few kicks into Terry. He was the father of the man who killed my brother. It was only right.

Ammonia hung around the air. Terry's trousers had been sopping wet when I landed my foot between his legs. I could get a diarrhoea niff too. Or it could have been just the smell of rain and a lot of dead fuckers. I thought we'd added a couple to the list before Terry launched into a low keen and Donie screeched and roared like a looper. Cribbing about his ribs and going on about brain damage.

The sole of Terry's shoe came in handy. Bumper struck a match off it and lit a Slim Panatella. The cigar lit first time despite the wind. Bumper bent down towards Terry. I waited for the glowing red nipple of light to extinguish itself in the man's eye. But Bumper just blew smoke in his face. He waited for Terry's racked cough to stop before he spoke to him.

—Tell your son, Fuck Dog or Master McGrath or Pedigree Chum or whatever he calls himself, tell him Bumper and Paul from Rathbawn are looking for him. Noelie Reilly's and Johnny Kelly's brothers. Tell him his family is getting off light. And tell him he ain't seen nothin' yet.

I almost tumbled backwards on to a heap of stones at the front wall of the cemetery but Bumper caught me in his arms.

It was a strange silence back in the car. Less the silence of not speaking than the silence of there being nothing to say. We both knew we'd moved the feud into a new set of rooms.

We'd gone too far. I knew that. There was no backing away from this now. We'd made a full-time job out of it. It was something that had to have a finish. You always want to turn back when you know you can't. That's when you realize all the different ways you could have acted. I realized on the way back to Rathbawn I didn't need to be where I was at the moment. I realized too I was stuck there.

Thick black muck clung to the bottom half of my Levis

and dried white shit was jammed in between the cleats on the soles of my shoes. We stopped outside a derelict creamery and the wind carried the flakes of shit in seven different directions as I banged the shoes against a wall. A bearded sailor looked benignly down on me from a Players Navy Cut sign twenty feet above my head.

We had broken some rule. Deffo. I told Bumper to fuck off when he asked if I wanted to drink some poitin in his house to round off the night. I took myself and my sense of doom back to the Park. He shouted after me.

—Who rattled your fucking cage, scobie? It's not like we killed anyone or anything, we only lucky-bagged out a few slaps.

He shouted more but between the wind and the hum of the generator from the fish factory the letters got broken up and scattered into the air like the incomplete pieces in the bottom of a tin of Alphabetti Spaghetti.

I knew the front door would be locked. But I pushed it all the same and swallowed hard when it didn't budge. I knew too the back window would be easy forced. I stayed facing the front door. Trying to think. Struggling to get things straight. I looked under the black rubber mat at the door even though there was no reason the front door key should be there for me. The mat sloughed off a stream of water when I lifted it. The water flowed down the path and the key glinted at me.

The key needed six goes to get into the lock. The first five left small gouges and scratches on the old lock. A comfort and a calm surrounded the opening click. Like the drift into sleep.

I slept all right. But Theresa Lawrence wouldn't quit my dreams.

Thirteen

Your Games, Your Rules

—The fags have me ruined. What the Vikings used do was saw out a man's breastbone, the sternum would be the medical terminology of words for it, and then they'd tear out his lungs and spread them out in front of him. They used call it the blood eagle. Only did you ever see what the fags does to your insides? If my lungs was spread out in front of me they'd look like a big flapping black raven.

It was the last thing the man in the white van said to me before he dropped me off near Bobby Sands Villas. I didn't recall a lot of the journey. Drunk again. And needful.

My face pressed so tight against Theresa's when I woke that my teeth brushed her nose when I yawned out some nerves.

—Mmmmmmmmmm.

Not exactly what she said. But

somewhat similar. I closed my mouth again and stayed where I was though there was nothing concrete to stop me moving. Nothing as concrete as Kerrie's leg strangling mine. Kerrie wouldn't like that line. She'd think using the word concrete about her leg was a dry jibe at her weight. Not that she had much. Her figure was good enough for a gallivant around Summer Bay any day of the week.

Funny how me and Theresa slept. Exactly straight out our full length. Turned into each other. Like we were petrified. You know, made of stone. Stuck together by sweat. A warm sweat instead of the cold one. My chest came away from Theresa's breasts with a sucking sound when I moved. I moved back in. Her toes pressed into my shins and slipped away. She opened her mouth. I breathed into it. She breathed back and opened her eyes. A joint chest billowed down the bed.

Theresa left her tongue in my mouth for a while. I flattened mine against the floor of my mouth so she could lick slowly and softly and casually around the walls of my cheeks and linger for a couple of moments on the cracks in my back teeth. She breathed deep. Her tongue was motionless. Like it was my mouth it belonged in.

Nobody had answered when I knocked on the front door. The early hours of the morning. The dark hours of the night. Between three and six. Coat-trailing after the last noise of the last people from the discos and the take-aways. Before light breaks open the envelope and unhappy people realize they won't be able to roll back to sleep. You can only look at the walls.

—Theresa, it's Paul Kelly, let me in.

A small light flicked on in her bedroom. I couldn't see but I felt visible. I twigged very late Theresa mightn't be there on her own. Some boyfriend could be there. Snoopy Giff could be there. The Kilfenora Ceili Band could be there.

—Paul, are you there?

—Yeah, I'm just outside the window, let me in please. I'll explain, you have to let me in.

On with the big light. Blink blink blink blink. Theresa Buddha-legged on the bed with a Pink Panther nightshirt pulled across her knees. A steak knife in her right hand. She left it back on the bedside locker. On top of the *Weekly World News*. She'd been sleeping on her own. Johnny's ironed denim shirt hung from a wire hanger balanced delicately on the chair at the bottom of the room.

—Fuck you, you fucking clown. Come in the back door. God, you're a pain in the hole.

I started to apologize. The bedroom light died and the back door opened while I stuttered and stammered some never-to-be-heard lie.

Something about Theresa's bare feet gave me a dull pain in the centre of my chest. Her Pink Panther melted into the multi-coloured map of the Cheeses of France on the wall behind her.

A glass of red wine was in my hand. A couple of minuscule cork traces hugged the edges of the glass. But you'd have to be a good barman to spot them. As good as me. Theresa turned a chair back to front. She sat with one leg either side of the back. Like Christine Keeler in the photo that turns up in the English papers the same time every year.

—It's only I have no place to stay, Theresa. I had to get out of Rathbawn.

—I don't want to hear about it.

—I'm sorry the way I scarpered the other morning.

—I'm not getting vexed about it, I'm just telling you I don't want to know anything about it.

—That's fair enough.

—That's fair enough. And the big sulky puss on you like the cat that got the caustic soda.

—I only want to sleep on the couch or any place. No strings attached.

Theresa bent her right leg and pulled it across to scratch the inside of her left knee.

—Oh, sure when you're here you might as well make yourself useful.

—............................

—And stop smirking. It's only I don't like the magazine I'm reading and there's a good bit of the night left yet.

—Yeah.

—Yeah. Look at you, you've a horn on you would drive an ass out of a sandpit.

It might be just enough to say that when I woke up and saw Theresa's freckles looking like brown tea splotched on a white tablecloth I didn't think of anything else for a few seconds.

It could be I saw the day ahead as being full of hours and minutes and seconds that would be too short. Instead of being one of those days when you look ahead from three o'clock and think how long life really is. All those hours like the Irish Mail trip to Holyhead.

I tried to pretend the arm I arced round Theresa could protect her from whatever set that Librium bottle rattling beside the bed.

She sprang up and looked out the back window to see if any of her washing had been nicked. There seemed no way to show her what I was thinking. There was nothing to say. All I could do was kneel on the floor and whisper the best prayer I could into her body. When her legs quivered she reached on to the chair at the bottom of the room and wrapped Johnny's shirt around her. A circus was in her voice when she skipped out the door.

—The two Kellys, ye're terrible, ye both do the same things.

I brought the clothes in off the line without being asked. This meant something. Or maybe it meant something else again. Theresa's things. Her knickers and bras flying gracefully in the view of ten trains each day. I buried my face in the heap of them for a second before I walked into the house.

More daytime TV. The boys sat quiet. I crumbled Club Goldgrain biscuits and dropped the pieces into Theresa's mouth. Her head in my lap. She looked up.

—I'll go over and get Martin Quilligan and we'll hit some place for the day.

Martin was the boy with the black beard. He lay across a couch in his caravan with a fedora pulled down over his eyes. *Going for Gold* on the box. Enough good furniture, glass and Delft around the caravan to fill four posh houses.

—Martin, how are you.

—Never better, lack, tell your friend if he breaks anything he'll pay for it one way or the other.

—Are you going any place today? It's a grand hot one.

—It is surely.

Theresa bit her bottom lip and pretended to be interested in two cut-glass decanters on a brown mahogany table. An antiques guide festooned with thumb marks sat beside them. I felt I should say something. Because of how I'd woken up that morning.

—I'm staying with Theresa and I'm planning to be around for a bit yet. Even if someone keeps trying to take the head off me with stones.

Martin flicked the hat off and left it on the floor. The insides of his eyes were opaque sheets of red. He put his hand out to me. I helped him up. He grimaced for a second while he tried to shift the weight off a gammy leg. I knew he was looking over my shoulder at Theresa. Something passed between them. A smile whipped through his lips for half a moment.

—Where will we go?

—Just to the local.

The van left Cordrum and passed through the little

villages that brought us into the next county. Two other vans came behind us. People looked in the windows of the vans and shook their heads dismissively when hiccuping tractors delayed us on the road.

The local perched on one side of a village green with a nursery-rhyme wishing-well in the middle. Twenty or thirty vans were parked outside it. Nissans, Hiaces, Lite-Aces. In a dead-straight line with plenty of space between them. Martin made sure to park his the same way before he saluted the two cops watching us.

The cops made a production out of looking at the tax disc when we locked the van. They waited till both doors were locked before they asked Martin for his driving licence and certificate of insurance or exemption. He smiled as he handed them over. Theresa kicked the kerb. I noticed how badly scuffed the toes of her white shoes were. The cops swapped the documents over and back between themselves.

—Martin Quilligan. It looks like him all right.

—It does, Gerry. Of course, they all look the same to me. It's all that oul inbreeding. Go on, son, and don't let us catch you making any trouble here.

Cactus Jacks. Great name for a jarring joint. The pub filled with whoops and hollers and the full sound of hands thumping off the broads of backs when we walked in. Theresa just smiled when people asked her what clan I was part of myself. A big grin that was smeared all over her face like someone else painted it there. She squeezed my hand. Martin jerked his thumb abruptly in my direction and whispered:

—Sham.

That dropped the volume of the conversation a couple of notches. Some of the older people moved away from me. But mainly the drink kept coming till the claps on the back sounded more like whip-cracks. I was surrounded by families in the middle of the floor. Lost. Someone with a bony finger tapped me on the shoulder.

—We're after buying a couple of bottles of whiskey down off the optic, come over and have a slug.

Martin was like he'd just woken up. The eyes were still red but they were jiving inside his skull. Doing the Huckle-buck even. He took a silver tankard out of his pocket, polished it with the sleeve of his jacket and handed it to me. Theresa laughed over the other side of the bar. The whiskey had me warmed up. Martin put his face close up to mine. Maybe trying to psych me. All I could think was if I went to bite his nose off he'd be in quare trouble.

—I want a word with you, sunshine.

—Word away, Martin, you oul hoor.

Martin took a deep breath and his eyes stopped rolling.

—I'm in good oul form, Mr Kelly, but I just have one bit of an oul warning to give you.

—What?

—Theresa Lawrence that's there. My sister-in-law. The finest woman I know. Mind her. She needs minding. All I want to say to you is mind that woman.

—Mind that woman.

That would be top of the list if you asked men their favourite thing to say to other men. It has everything. Myself and Martin heard Theresa's bubbling, swooping laugh splash around Cactus Jacks. The laugh of someone no one would ever need to mind. No one would be able to.

A set of swing-door squeals announced the cops. One lad made a show out of flat-footing round to the side door. He would have been trampled if any gang had wanted to make a run for it. No one heeded the cops. It was like the West Indian pubs on the Brixton front line. Business as usual. No big deal. Your games, your rules. The landlady stayed serving and didn't look at the filth. The main man had inspector's pips on the uniform. You didn't see them out that often.

—Excuse me, miss, but I was talking to you, said the inspector to the landlady even though he hadn't been.

The landlady picked up an Irish stew recipe dishcloth and swabbed the bone-dry counter in front of the inspector. She hummed an Abba tune. The inspector looked around and shook his head. Hard. A couple of the cops checked the jacks and came back shaking their heads as well.

—Right. We're looking for some people who were involved in an altercation in Ballinasloe. One of them was stabbed in the face and he'd be bleeding fairly heavily. Joyces or Maughans, did anyone here see any of them?

The sound of talk started up. The pub was loud again within a few seconds. The landlady stuck her elbows up on the counter.

—You know damn well that none of those people drinks here. Ballinasloe is a long way away. Did anyone tell you they were here?

The cops at the swing doors stopped a couple of women and kids from leaving the pub. The inspector fiddled with his tie and turned away from the counter. He sucked his teeth.

—We thought they might be here. After all, there's not many pubs where they'd get served. We'll see how smart you are next month when your licence is up for renewal.

—Dickheads.

The word followed the filth to the door and stuck to their backs.

We left soon after. Theresa rubbed her hands together a lot. A few yards away from the van we noticed all the broken glass on the footpath. Two men in brown leather jackets hammered the side of Martin's van with car jacks. They weren't that steady on their feet and didn't see Martin till he was on top of them. One of them managed to ditch his jack and boot it up the town. The other slipped as he tried to get away. He swung the jack at Martin from the ground and grazed his knee. Martin stamped down on his hand and kicked him hard into the face.

The man rolled slowly backwards. Away from Martin. He was well on it but he was soberer than Martin who hit off the side of the van and fell when he tried to land a second kick. The leather jacket struggled to his feet and put his hand up to his face. His palm was pure red when he took it down. He looked like he'd been hand-painting. Martin rolled around on the ground with his shoulder busted. The man spat down at him and waved a fist into the air.

—Knackers, ye dirty, smelly knackers, keep out of our town.

A few more people were out of the pub now. The man would have got away in plenty of time if Theresa hadn't taken a screwdriver out of her pocket and jabbed him in the elbow. He stepped back and fell over Martin. Martin stumbled up and kicked him a few times in the ribs. The street was full now. A couple of squads moved down towards the pub. Followed by a group of men led by the guy who'd dropped the jack and run off. Theresa threw the screwdriver away. Her face was gone pure white.

—What could I do, what could I do?

What she did then was bundle Martin into the van and take the keys off him. The cops had a good look at our van but let us go. A few punches and kicks from the locals added to the dents. Theresa leaned over the steering wheel and kept driving. A squad picked up on our tail just outside the town. The lights shone in our back window and clicked on and off for a while before the cops turned back.

Theresa bought a take-away for supper and rolled Martin into bed. When we sat down in the house it almost seemed that . . . It almost seemed that . . . It almost seemed that. But I can't say it and when the thought poked through the skin the phone rang and dragged Theresa out of my arms and into her hall. She shouted it was for me. I knew there would be no stop now.

—Hello, me oul segosha. You're very hard gotten hold of these days. Did you ever think of hiring an agent?

—Bumper.

—Not anybody else. Listen, I'm in the bar of the Cordrum Arms. See me here as quick as you can.

Bumper was hard seen in his big wicker chair. At the front of the lobby. A torn poster on the wall above reception told us the Cordrum Arms Hotel's famous Irish cabaret took place tonight.

The concreted remains of the canal spur pulled chaotic sounds from the suspension of Bumper's latest car. People had given up living in the Harbour Cottages years before I went to England. Now they were back. The memory of Big Bird Robbo cutting tape with ceremonial scissors hung over the crafts centres in the first four cottages. We stopped at the fifth one. Bumper ducked in the low front door. It was open. *Match of the Day* blared from the sitting-room. Bumper decided to come back outside and knock on the front door.

—Manners. He's a funny oul fucker.

The funny oul fucker was out in a shot when he heard the knock. His lazy right eye circumnavigated the gaff and fixed on the baseball bat inside the door before he shook hands with Bumper. He looked coiled. The way Bumper did sometimes.

—All right, Bumper, mate. Kathleen, can you bring us in a few cups of tea? Or would you like a few bottles of beer, lads? You Irish, you like your beer, don't you?

—Tea is grand.

—Fair enough. Graaand, yeah, heh-heh, graaand, it's the way you say it.

The voice brought me back down the Old Kent Road to

234

that time of night when home was one alternative and Casualty the other.

We sat down. The little Englishman lay across the couch. Me and Bumper sat on two ludicrous beanbags that unbalanced and toppled over every couple of minutes. Our host chuckled to himself. Pointedly. A frightened-looking woman in a pastel-coloured tracksuit brought in a massive tray of tea, sandwiches and Jacob's Mikado biscuits. The biscuits had melted and congealed into a couple of large, sticky wedges. The Englishman dug his fingers into them and scooped out a large lump of jam, sponge and biscuit. He chewed it off his hand and was getting ready to speak when a six-year-old kid bounced in the door with an open colouring book in her hand.

—Nick, Nick, look what I done.

Nick reached his hand out, took the page from the book and flittered it into tiny pieces before hitting the kid a crack across the face. The child was going to cry but the woman in the tracksuit dragged her out of the room. Then she came back in and poured the tea. We heard the child outside in the hall. The stifled sound of a kid not crying when it needs to. The saddest sound of all. Nick banged his mug against the table and didn't notice the scalding tea flowing over his wrist.

—I fucking told you to keep your daughter out of here when I'm doing business, Kathleen. I fucking told you. She makes me nervous, she's doing my fucking head in, you know how I get these fucking headaches, just keep her out of my fucking way.

Bumper whispered in the guise of a cough:

—This is why they call him Nutty Nick.

I concentrated on a damp green patch between the ceiling and a stone wall.

—You have the oul gun, Nick?

—I have. The oul gun, heh-heh, the way you says that. I can let you have a new one for £500 or a used one for £150. You know the hassle with the old one, it's got a history so it's up to you to worry about that.

—We're not planning on getting caught, the old gun will do, said Bumper.

Nick jumped off the couch and walked out of the room. We heard a rusty bolt being slid back, saw a light come on in the back yard and listened to the metallic rooting sound of his search. I got a shiver. Kathleen stood in the doorway with her mouth open but not a word coming out.

A tin was in Nick's paw when he came back. According to the inscription it once held Danish Butter Biscuits. I tried to remember if I'd ever eaten them but my mouth stayed clear like it does when I eat cucumber.

—This place is a bastard to heat. It's 'cause of that old jingle-jangle Royal Canal. I love those Paddy songs. Here you go, Bumper, mate, this should do the trick.

He stuck the gun on the coffee table with the barrel pointing towards Gary Lineker on the television. It wasn't that big really. Only there was a sort of a hum off it. Expectancy. Like a shiny knife, like a needle, like a full bottle beside the bed at half eight in the morning. Two notches burned or gouged into the handle.

—Smith and Wesson .38, my gun of choice, my son. Decommissioned to me by a mate in the Six Counties or Ulster or whatever you is calling them these days. In good nick.

—It looks well.

—It does, don't it. It's funny, it's done people on both sides.

I half expected the gun to blush with pride.

—The job should be Oxo with that, Nick.

Bumper opened the biscuit tin before he started the car.

—You're taking the gun, Paul.

236

—I'm not. I never used a handgun in me life. The only thing I ever shot was rabbits when I was fourteen.

—You are. It's easier than shooting rabbits. All you have to do is walk up behind Giff, stick this just behind his ear and pull the trigger. I'll be there with you, I might do it meself yet.

—Why can't you hang on to the gun?

—Because rasher squad is always searching my place for stolen stuff. It's handier in your house. Just keep it some place cool.

—I'm not taking it.

—Don't get this way with me now. I'm after paying Nick fair spondulics for that gun. I never asked you for a red cent and I wouldn't take one off you. I'm only asking you to mind this for a couple of days.

—A couple of days?

—Cross my heart and hope to die, pudding. There's only Giff left. I reckon this stuff about a big boss man in Abbeytown is all shit. Come on, I'm fed up with this as well. A couple of shots and we've killed the man who killed our brothers.

—Yeah. OK. Hunky-dory.

I felt ashamed when I got home. There was a reason for this. A real reason. A good reason. My brother Johnny not to be dead for nothing. Something had to be different. Things couldn't not change. It'd look like I wasn't trying. I rang Theresa. I could tell she was waiting up. I said there was nothing wrong. I'd be back tomorrow afternoon but I had to go home for the night. She said OK. I went to stow the gun.

Lights were on in the kitchen. I went straight to Kaya's bedroom. She looked asleep. But she started babbling when I sat on the bed. She tried to sit up but flopped down again. The babbling ended with a painful intake of breath. A reversed shriek. I rocked her a few times.

—OK, pet. You OK?

—Yeah.

—Come on, pet. You'll be all right. Are you sure you'll be all right?

—Yeah ... It's just ... I thought that things ... I thought...

If her sleep was the same as her mother's she wouldn't remember waking up at all. The blinds threw shadows like truncated prison bars down one side of her face.

Fourteen

A Stroll in the Oul Bamboo Gardens

The shopping centre carpark was filling quick but they hadn't got round to parking in the handicapped spaces yet. I sat on a bench and rested my head between my knees. The black tarmac looked solid. So solid you couldn't imagine that one day it wouldn't be there.

A blue Honda Civic pulled up in front of my bench. The cop or whatever he was who'd played cat's cradle in the barracks rolled down the window. A pair of red furry dice hung suggestively over his head.

—Mr Kelly, how're ya doin'. Do you want an oul lift at all?

—I'm OK.

—You don't look OK to me. You look fucked. I can see the smell rising off you. Come on, you could do with a seat home.

—Fuck off.

He opened the door on the driver's

side. A car came up behind him. It couldn't get past. The driver hooted the horn. The cop or whatever looked back at him and shook a thick fist. The driver didn't hoot a second time. He just sat there drumming his fingers against the dashboard. It made me think of the start of the *Lone Ranger* music.

—Get in to fuck or I'll kick you senseless. Don't think I wouldn't.

I knew he would. His shoes were shined up so much you could see his reflection in them. The air in the car was clogged up with the stink of stale air-freshening devices. The plastic was still on the seats. An unopened packet of Polo mints rolled around the dashboard. The cop snapped it in two and offered me half.

—It's OK, really.

—No, I insist. Really. The mints might take the smell off your breath. It smells like you've been muff-diving a priest's housekeeper.

—Am I being arrested?

—What are you on about? I'm not acting as a Special Branch man here. I'm just a friend who happens to be giving you a lift.

—So I can get out of the car if I want to.

—Don't be like that. Or I'll break your back.

The cop didn't say anything when we were in the car. He just sang along to a couple of corny C. & W. classics.

Something to do with closed doors and hair hanging low played when we passed through the old demesne gates and drove into the Forest Park. A young fella in a wooden hut asked us for admission money at the bottom of the hill. The cop waited for me to check my pockets before he paid in for both of us.

—Don't tell me I never do anything for you, Paul.

We stuck the car in the carpark. This one was nearly empty. We walked up the hill to where Lord Rathbawn lived before the forces of anti-imperialism burned down his big house where the local people had been forced to labour for the oppressor for so many years. Now they didn't have to take the cursed Saxon Shilling and they could work for Abrakebabara or Rathbawn Meats or the Korean mob who owned the video-tape factory out on the industrial estate.

No. No more Rathbawn House.

The cop was blowing a bit when we got to the top of the hill. He lit a smelly half-corona with leaves falling out every side of it.

—Smoke?

—No, I don't.

—You're missing out, I'm telling you. These are something else. What sort of a country is it when they replace Rathbawn House with something like this? It's a fucking monstrosity. Well, needs must something or other. I can't remember the end of it but I think it's good.

—Something to do with the devil.

—You're the boy would know.

Sometimes the gates of the grey concrete tower were locked halfway up. They weren't this day. We reached the top and looked down at the lake, the Forest Park and the town. A pair of teenagers in swimming gear clambered all over each other on a secluded part of the lakeshore. OK, a relatively secluded part. The sight made me uneasy. But we both watched.

—It's some view from up here. You can see the whole town.

—But why would you want to, Paul?

—It's not the worst town.

I knew from his accent he wasn't local. So he had no right to agree with what I thought myself.

—Are you a political man yourself, Paul?

—I haven't an ounce of interest in it.

—That's about the most political way you can be. In order

for evil to triumph it is only necessary for good men to do nothing. Who said that?

—Edmund Burke.

—I thought you'd think Edmund Burke is the name of a supermarket chain.

—I know that because it's one of two things crabby cunts like you always use in letters to the papers. The other one is 'I disagree with what you say but I will defend to the death your right to say it.'

—Voltaire.

—I thought you'd think Voltaire was the name of an Andy Williams record.

—I'm getting vertigo. Come on, we'll go down.

The Ice House is where they used store the meat for the big house. To keep it fresh. A sort of an escape tunnel ran from the big house to the Ice House. Stalactites hung down from the roof. Little ones. The cop slipped a couple of times in the tunnel but didn't hit the ground. The Ice House stays cool on the hottest days. We climbed the steps and looked down into the big pit.

The oul fella used lift me up on to the railing of the Ice House. I could look down and think what it would be like in the big pit. How impossible it would be to get out. I would sit on the railing with only my father's arm around me to stop me falling. I wanted to bring Kaya to the Ice House.

—I'm Special Branch. Do you know what that means?

—Yere a sort of a law to yereselves.

—It means you get called a Brancher bastard by little fuckers with moustaches who spit at you when you arrest them for selling Easter lilies without a permit.

—Groovy job.

—The fucking North should be cut off from the rest of this island and towed out to some place near the North Pole.

—What about Dana?

—You don't know how much you owe people like me.

They were going to take over this country, all that mob, the Provies, the Irps and so on. They would have only for us.

—No, they weren't.

—How would you know? You weren't out of short trousers then. The politicos told us to stop them. We hated it. I was as republican as the next man. I'm Irish. But we did our job. Harassing the cunts, kicking the shite out of them, helping them fall down stairs so they'd sign confessions. That put them out of the way.

—Why are you telling me about all this shite?

—I don't know. Because you're stuck here and because you have to listen to me and because in my own good time I'm going to tell you who was behind the killing of your brother. The big man at the top.

—Who?

—I said in my own good time. This is all important for you to hear. It'll give you a valuable overview. In the end, anyways, we broke their fucking hearts, we wiped them out down here. But then the politicians got cold feet and started listening to the bleeding hearts and giving out about the way we treated those cunts. They turned on us and now we're the bad boys.

—Who killed Johnny?

—Do you know what, I'd love a stroll in the oul Bamboo Gardens.

It was always easy to get lost in the Forest Park Bamboo Gardens. All those lovely thin bamboo clumps looking like each other. So many entrances and exits. Positively the best place to play the spiffing war games myself and Johnny used be into. Myself and Johnny.

The cop snapped off sticks of bamboo as we walked. His body trembled. His eyes misted up. I almost expected him to break down and start pounding the ground with his hands. It was baked hard and would give off an impressive thumpy, echoing sound.

—We should have got medals, you know. For what we did. But no one else saw the thing as clear as we did.

—Who killed Johnny?

—Keep walking.

The Bog Gardens used be my favourite place in the Forest Park. Funny, really, because I'm not a flowers and plants man and the one time I went to Kew with Lydia I was bored stiff and she said I had no sense of beauty and I said look at yourself in the mirror, my love, and you'll see you're wrong about that.

Perhaps it was the colours. Or the wooden tree stumps in the path. It could have been the rickety wooden bridge you crossed to enter the Gardens. The cop started talking when we got on to the bridge.

—How and ever, Ireland is fucked and so is your poor wee brother and I met you to tell who arranged for himself and young Reilly to get the tar.

—Who?

He paused for dramatic effect. Big into the amateur drama was the bould Branch man. You could see him running around the stage of a parish hall trying to get the neighbour's wife out of the bedroom before the vicar arrived for tea.

Or maybe it was mindfucks he was into. I'd say he was some crack when he turned up with a confession and a biro after you'd gone twenty hours without a wink of sleep.

—Cathal O'Hagan.

—Who?

—In my game everyone knows Cathal O'Hagan. We'd go back a long oul stint, meself and Cathal. I got him three years when he was only a gossan back in '72 for trying to kill an RUC man up around the border.

—He's a Provo?

—He's a bollocks. But he was never much of a joiner. That's why they call him the Lone Wolf. He was supposed to be part of some splinter group from the INLA. It had a big long name with the words revolutionary and workers in it, which is a gas seeing as Cathal never did a hand's turn in his life. His fellow freedom fighters referred to Cathal's gang as the Fermanagh Balubas. He killed most of the other lads in it in the end.

—What had he to do with Johnny? Johnny had no interest in that sort of crack.

—O'Hagan is doing a bit in the crime line at the moment and you know how thieves fall out. But he might have had your brother killed for the crack or anything. He's not all in the game, the same Cathal. He blew up a pub once because they barred him. I remember him kidnapping some poor unfortunate bank manager a few years back. He chiselled off the man's little fingers and sent them to the family when they were dragging their heels over the ransom. We could have got him then. I wanted to set up a bit of an ambush so we could shoot him dead in self-defence. But they wouldn't have it so he got back to the North and did six years there for something else.

—What is he doing down here?

—What indeed?

Something about the Forest Park Gazebo makes you feel they built the peace and quiet in. Nailed it somewhere in the domed roof. Or sprinkled it all around the circular floor. I heard water moving round the lake and the clean clicking of the tips on Brancher Bastard's shoes as he paced up and down.

—The Wolf seems to have jacked in the armed struggle since he got out of the quare place the last time. He's living on an estate in Abbeytown, running drugs. Or is it pushing drugs? I can never remember. He sells dirty videos, lends money, works protection rackets, makes a crust the best way he knows.

—Why don't you arrest the fucker?

—Technicalities. We don't have the evidence. Giff did

the last couple of jobs for him. The Lone Wolf is on the go a bit long now, in fairness, to get done by small-town cops. He's a hard man to track down.

—You know a lot about this gent.

—I do. I take a personal interest in him. I know every Tuesday morning at half ten he goes into the Chieftain Bar down from the power station in Abbeytown to have a couple of cups of coffee and a bit of a chat with his mates. He doesn't come out too often, you see, he's too crafty. He keeps a man on the door of the Chieftain to see it stays locked.

—Where does he live?

—He sleeps with a gun under his pillow in a different room every night. But if you were to let on you were a rep and someone provided you with a nice car with a brewery logo you'd get in the door of the Chieftain and the Wolf wouldn't be silly enough to have a gun handy in the pub.

—What's in it for you?

—He deserves to die. Think of your brother. The Wolf thinks he's a big shot but he's fucking not, you know. He just thinks he is, so he does. The car'll be parked just down from your mammy's house the morning after tomorrow.

—What am I supposed to do?

Click. Click. Click. Click. Clickety-click. Click.

—I know ye bought that gun from thon English prick in Cordrum. I give you my word you can go into that pub and shoot our friend and there won't be a word said. I give you my word right. Cross my heart and hope to die. All will be looked after.

Make-your-mind-up time.

I nodded my head. He nodded back. I smiled. He smiled.

Special Branch cleared away a little circle in the dust on the window and peered out at the lake like it was an edgy animal poised to attack him.

Silence again in the car. He only spoke when he dropped me off at the War of Independence monument.

—You should go out to the Forest Park more often. It's a marvellous facility to have on your doorstep.

I felt like a kid again when the car disappeared around the corner. Was there an instruction manual somewhere on how to be a man? Some guide to the wiring system? Some City and Guilds certificate? Because there were times I felt like I was only playing at it. Somebody somewhere knew I hadn't made the cut.

Lydia.

It ended the sunny day when Lydia talked Vinnie into letting her bring Kaya out in the pram. She smiled a lot and shamed him into it by talking a lot about trust. And about the old days.

The cops arrived back with her that evening.

Kaya.

She'd been left in the pram on the North Peckham estate. Four floors up beside a disused lift shaft. Her mum went off to score some smack. Some young bucks heard Kaya bawling and screaming and rang the nick.

Vinnie said he read that kids don't remember things that happen when they're that young. Kaya was hardly one year old. Hardly. But that day ended me with Lydia.

She came back to the pub for the last time four days later. She asked me for money. A couple of thousand quid would do. It was only fair, Paul. Profits were good and she was part of the management team. You always say, she said, we're a team. No, I said, not after what you did to our daughter. She spat in my face then and called me names I'd never heard her use before. They sounded like they were on loan from someone else's mouth.

—You're only a fucking child, Paul.

She took a running jump into the car outside. The driver was a head from Liverpool who'd done an eight-stretch for armed robbery. He stabbed Sean through the heart two weeks later after a row over nominating a pocket for the eight in a game of pool. I changed the locks and took up sleeping in the afternoons instead of at night. In shreds of sleep like the little flakes of left-over tobacco at the bottom of the pouch that are never enough to make even one small rollie.

Vinnie and myself spent two whole days on the batter a while later when O'Neill's brother opened a big new pub in Walthamstow named after a racehorse. Near the end of the second day Vinnie told me he'd seen Lydia standing in the doorway of a porno cinema in King's Cross. Her thin legs shivering in a pair of black mesh tights full of holes. The Arkle, I think, was the name of the pub. Or it might have been the Monksfield. The Dawn Run sort of rings a bell.

All I felt that time was relief because I knew she wouldn't be coming back.

Fifteen

Goat, the Goat, Goat, the Goat

Nothing seemed real in the Imperial Hotel. Imitation logs burned for ever in a Rathbawn grate. The only presence from the Park was a lounge girl or an occasional harassed red face popping out the kitchen door for a few cooling seconds. The Imperial was in another world. The perfect place to go if you wanted to forget you'd agreed to kill a man.

—Pint of Guinness and a Jemmy and ice, please.

God, it was true. They did give you a receipt with every drink. And the Crosbys were still too mean to put in a paging system so the lounge girls had to do the rounds of the big bar asking lonely drunken reps is that your name and if it is you're wanted on the phone. Lonely men like the one the other side of the bar waving and shouting at me.

—Paul Kelly, Paul Kelly, come over here.

Except this lonely man was scrap mogul Eddie Clyne. He unfurled a fist-thick roll of twenties kept together by a brown elastic band, extracted one smelling of new leather and old tobacco and shouted another round. Whiskey and porter arrived for me with a bottle of Ballygowan that Eddie poured into a glass with ice and a rindy lemon slice.

I twitched when something like the hoofbeats of the ghost riders in the sky clattered over our heads.

—It's the line-dancing upstairs, said a lounge girl with a yellow scrunchie in her hair.

She pointed to the poster on the pillar in front of us. 'The Denim and Lace Country Club with DJ Cotton-Eye Joe. The most fun you can have with your boots on.'

The devil going down to Georgia just over his head put Eddie off for a few seconds. He kept telling me how successful we both were until he suddenly stopped and tried to melt into the pillar quivering under the stomps of two hundred line-dancers.

Because who came across the floor towards us and scutched civil servants out of the way to remind them why they'd refused to move to Rathbawn unless they got a promotion, only Clinger and him moving in a heavy stagger like the sub-mariner emerging from the depths with seaweed tangled round his legs.

—Ah, well, yes, y'know, that sort of thing, said Eddie and studied the Denim and Lace poster with great interest.

A lot of white showed in Clinger's eye. Like you'd see on an oul mad horse. He steadied himself with a hand that left a black smudge on Eddie's light-grey slacks. Eddie pushed his hand away and left it resting on the back of his chair.

—Clinger. Go home, boss, don't be a mong boy. Everything is going to be all right. Go home to your woman and your child. Come on, I'm sorry, I'll drive you down.

Eddie looked like he thought Clinger was taking the piss,

though from the smell of Clinger he hadn't taken it very far away. I put an empty glass up on the counter. Clinger stopped gurgling and looked at me before letting a roar out. A big, savage roar. And again. Pure pain. The overhead fiddling and banjo playing stopped. Clinger screamed:

—*Nooooooooooooooooooowaaaaaaaa. Nooooooooooo.*

He pushed Eddie. Eddie slipped off his stool which followed down in semi-slow motion and fell on top of him. Clinger ran for the door with Eddie's plea following.

—Get him, Paul. Please.

I ran after Clinger but he had a head start on me and made up more ground because fallen people and chairs littered his wake. He was at the far end of the foyer by the time I got out of the bar.

—Clinger, stop, Jesus, I'm your friend.

He turned and looked at me and yowled again before he drew his arm back and smashed it through a glass door. He pulled it out quickly. The red looked unreal, like ketchup or some sort of soup. Thick splotches stood out on the thread-bare welcome mat he crossed to get to the door.

More glass broke. More people screamed. Clinger's scream mixed with a choir of high-pitched female shrieks. They weren't much less panicky. A thick lump of tinted brown glass flew to one side of my head as I got out the door.

Clinger was pegging beer barrels through the windows of the Imperial Hotel. Pegging them through the opaque surface and roaring.

—I never done any harm to anyone. I never done no harm to no one.

I walked towards him and he left down a barrel. It rolled obligingly into the road and caused the first squad car to brake suddenly. He ran towards me and hugged me. In a kind of a desperate way. The way Kaya had after we'd talked about where you go when you die. My cheek was wet with

Clinger's tears. I felt the blood funnel out of his arm and tickle the back of my neck. He was sobbing. The sound of sirens nearly drowned him out.

—It broke my heart, Paul.

—It'll be all right, Clinger, you'll be all right.

His heart was broke. You could see that in the white part of his eye. He said it one more time and the next second the cops dragged him away from me. A cop shouted that Clinger had bitten him in the chest and the next thing Clinger was down on the ground with about a dozen of them laying into him. A sergeant came over to me and said:

—It's under control, sir, there's nothing to worry about.

There's nothing to worry about. That's a good one. Did he not think I'd know if there wasn't?

Theresa was resting on one elbow when I opened my eyes the next morning. Looking at me. I woke up properly when she leaned over to pick up something beside the bed and her breasts slid across my chest.

—Drink some of this Diet Coke, Paul. I thought you might want a supeen of it when you came back to life.

—You're awful good.

—Awful good in me fuck. I wanted a kiss good morning and I didn't fancy eating those flakes off the inside of your gob.

We had a kiss good morning. But it was more than a kiss we wanted. Both of us. Yeah. Both of us. Because we were a both that morning. The thought that either of us would be able to look at the other from the outside was as silly as the position we ended in. It took an awkwarder reach than usual to cradle Theresa but now it was all I thought of. My shoulder joint cracked. Theresa raised her tongue against the sole of my foot. Silent. Still. Rare for it to be like this.

Triangles of toast slotted neatly into a sterling silver rack on the table.

—Well domestic.

—Martin gave it to me. It's very nice.

I better explain something before I go any further. In case the wrong idea is got. It's just that I'm going to use the word love soon. But that's a whatyoumaycallit coincidence. I'm not using the word because I was sat at that wobbly table with myself and Theresa picking slices of toast from silver. It has nothing to do with the way Theresa dabbed a wet finger into the small pile of crumbs on the table and stuck it into her mouth. It's nothing to do with that. God's honest truth.

The day after the cops landed Kaya home I went down the North Peckham myself. Just to see. I tried to work out where the pram had been left. Where Lydia would have been standing. What view she would have had of her only child. Did she look back? Or did she just turn on her heel and run away from the pram in case she'd change her mind? The sound of the crying must have been tough. Nine months and all those hours of pain in King's College Hospital. For what?

So there I was clomping through this architect's revenge when I saw sprayed on a wall in four-foot-high letters DEBBIE WILKINS LOVES LAMBERT JOSEPH.

I looked at it for a few seconds and thought how much handier they were getting with the spray cans. Then I looked at it again. And this time I saw it. I thought, yeah, she does too. And he did too because underneath in smaller but neater pink letters was LAMBERT JOSEPH LOVES DEBBIE WILKINS.

Shit smeared along the bottom of the wall. A gaggle of needles lying nearby. But you still had love in four-foot-high letters. I started seeing the walls all the time from then on. In Stonebridge Park, in the dodgy subway at the head of Lea

Bridge Road, in the Bullring, near Lincolns Inn Fields. And in Colmcille Park. Someone always loved someone else on the wall. I told myself that even in Rwanda or that city in Mozambique where people live in abandoned zoo cages someone carves two names on a tree or abstractedly traces them in the sand with a big toe.

One night I was staggering home through Elephant and Castle Tube when I saw a couple of young headcases running away after kicking the shit out of a couple of old winos. The man lay up against the wall with his face battered in. The woman was wailing.

—Look what they done to my man, look what these fucking bastards done to my man, come back ye cunts, you'll be all right darling, you'll be all right, get the fucking ambulance, ye dog's abortions ye, you'll be OK pet, I love you.

Someone probably loved the headcases too.

I still don't think that has anything to do with myself and Theresa singing along with the radio all the way over to Rathbawn in a van Martin Quilligan loaned us.

—I think it might be taxed and I'd say you might be insured on it and you'll hardly meet a shade this hour of the morning anyways. And if you do, tell them the policy definitely covers you in England and that you'll get in touch with the Guardian Royal Exchange because they say it covers you here and all.

The key was still under the mat.

Theresa tripped in after me. Tommy and Simon hiding their faces in the folds of her coat. There had been no need to bring her but less to leave her behind. I checked the kitchen for Mam. I always checked there first.

Kaya gazed sternly at a quiz show. Her toddler hi-tops hung halfway between the settee and the carpet. It didn't seem all that long ago when I couldn't get up on the settee at the first attempt. Because I was small, not because I was drunk. All the lights came on in Kaya's face when she saw us. Because I was back. Or as likely because I had brought new people with me. She could be a right little show-off, the same girl.

—All right, champ.

—All right, Dad. Where you been?

—Business, pet. Out on business.

—Business, hmmm, well, don't let it happen again, she said and rolled the new phrase blissfully around her mouth.

Her cheery witch's cackle made Simon take his face out of his mother's coat and his thumb out of his streaming mouth. Kaya took him in with a superior interest. The little hi-tops swung back and forward. She had a confidence none of the other Park kids had. And she hadn't lost any of it in Rathbawn. Yet. There are a lot of yets about. I hadn't killed the Lone Wolf yet.

—This is my friend Theresa, Kaya.

—Hello, Theresa.

—Hello, Kaya, you have a lovely name.

—Thank you. It's the only one I got.

Kaya burst into giggles before looking at her thumb and pondering whether to suck it shyly or not. She decided not.

—Where's Granny, champ?

—She's just gone in to Missus Greer. She's only going to be there a bit.

I picked Kaya up. Amazing the weight of a child of four compared to the same kid at two. The march of time and all that and one day they beat you at arm wrestling.

—Come on, kids, we're going.

We were walking past Donoghue's when I decided the kids would like minerals and crisps. Joe put up the first round. Ozzie Small staggered across the bar with his legs looking bent twice below the knees and tried to tap us. We were looking in our pockets when Joe let a roar and Ozzie ran for the door. He still sang the same song.

—That man was very smelly.

—Don't say that, Kaya, it's not very nice.

—But he was, Dad, he smelt like wee-wees.

—Don't say it, Kaya, it's personal.

—But I'm a person, ain't I, Dad?

No reason or right for dumping Kaya with Mam if you looked at it. Even if I was going to drag her around to Donoghue's every day I should keep her with me. As her father. As a team. Which is what we always had been despite it all. She had to be with me. For both our sakes. If I lost that idea I was splashing around altogether. Splish splosh. Glug glug glug. Drown.

Theresa played one potato, two potato, three potato, four, with Kaya. If you did it in reverse you could call it a Great Famine commemoration and get a massive grant.

—Do I see a frown? Turn it upside down.

I turned around quickly but it was young Simon who had the puss on him. Kaya smiled away with those worrying teeth. Almost a shine coming off her. People should be that happy. My daughter could show them how. I kissed her on the cheek and told her I'd be back in ten minutes and didn't even bother to add the usual rider about being a good girl because it just seemed impossible she could be anything else. At that moment I could see myself and Kaya and Theresa. And? And? I could. For a split second.

The key was in my pocket. Mam hoovered the sitting-room furiously like she always did when she was wobbly. We learnt early on that a lot of Brasso, Jif or Shake 'n' Vac moving at high speed meant a worrying day and Tracey sending us out to play. Some phone-in was on the radio but the asthmatic puffing of the ancient Nilfisk meant you heard tones instead of words. Johnny had promised to get her a new vacuum cleaner but he died the day before he was supposed to buy it.

—Mam.

Hoover, hoover and hoover and bash the nozzle against the side of the fireplace.

—Mam, please.

—What? I'm busy.

—Do you want me to make a cup of tea then, Mam?

—OK.

—Where are the teabags?

—Oh, listen, you'll make a mess out of lighting the gas and you'll scatter everything looking for those teabags. I'll do it myself.

—No, Mam, sit down for once. You don't work behind a bar without learning how to make a decent cup of tea.

—Well, there's no need to take the head off me.

—Ah, Mam.

I brought her in biscuits and everything and even wrapped the teapot in this huge cosy I found at the back of the press beside the Roche Fives. Mam got a good laugh out of the big orange cosy smothering the small teapot. She enjoyed that. She would have been great at laughing given the opportunities to practise it.

—I don't want to fall out with you, Paul, but I'm very fond of my little granddaughter and I heard you have her below in Donoghue's with that knacker Johnny used be seeing.

—Theresa's all right.

—You know nothing, Paul. When you're my age you'll know people just can't go around the place doing what they want.

She broke a little corner off a hard gingernut and ground it into dust on the plate with the flat of her right thumb.

—She's not a bad girl, Mam. She was very attached to Johnny.

—You could do better than hanging around with that one. She's a pure-bred tinker. I hear you can get the smell of the camp off her still.

—I know what she is, Mam. When you're beyond and you come back these differences don't seem to be the same big deal any more.

—But you could do better, Paul. I didn't mind you not coming home or writing once I knew you were doing so well. But I don't want you ending up mixing with the same sort of people that Johnny did. You were better off than him. You always knew what you were at, don't get mixed up with some sketch that's not long in from under the canvas.

—Theresa is very good with Kaya. They're hitting it off like old pals below in Donoghue's.

—What sort of a woman is lodged abroad in a pub at this hour? The tinkers is inferior people and you're letting yourself down.

There's points when nothing can be said. So nothing is what you say. Mam looked sadly into her cup of tea and poked her finger through the cold crust on top of it. Some of it attached to her nail and slid slowly down the side of the cup.

—I'll go then, Mam. I'll be back in a bit though.

The phone rang. I walked past it first and opened the door. Then I leaned back and picked up the receiver. Providence, as the man says.

—Hello. Hello, Paul.

Kerrie's voice kicked the front door shut.

—Hello, Kerrie.

—Hi. How's tricks?

—Oh, tricks are grand.

Crackle. Crackle. And the faint hint of someone else's conversation peeking in from a crossed line.

—I've been trying to ring you for ages but no one ever seems to answer the phone.

—I've been out and about quite a bit.

—Are you OK, Paul? Are you looking after yourself?

—I'm OK. It's good to hear from you.

The sound of my voice came back off the walls. It sounded like my voice. It didn't always.

—It's good to hear you too. Everyone's been asking for you. Mr O'Neill says you can take another couple of weeks off if you want to.

—I don't know if I will or not. I'm confused.

—I know you are. I understand. I miss you very much. Everyone does. You know, you haven't had a holiday in two years.

—Sure I'm on a permanent holiday.

—When are you coming back? The bed's too big without you.

—Soon. You sound great. Well, you don't, you sound like you've been up all night chug-a-lugging spirits but it's just, you know, your voice.

—Thanks. You know, everything is going to be OK, Paul. When you get back we'll make a fresh start. Everyone says they think you'll pull through. Mr O'Neill says the pub is still going brilliant.

—Do you honestly think everything will be all right. Seriously?

—It will, Paul. You know it will. Maybe we can even start some sort of a real life together, me and you and Kaya.

—Maybe you're right. Isn't there some sort of saying about if wishes were fishes then poor men would be Captain Birdseye? Or is that just a cod? Is Vinnie there?

—He's downstairs.

—Put him on for a couple of ticks will you. 'Bye. I miss you. I really do.

—I love you.

She might do. I definitely missed her though I'd run every sort of a memory of my life through my head for a week without thinking of her.

Things you could think about Kerrie.

Her taking those long steps of hers with the rucksack

slung over her shoulder and her mate Kim with her and them asking were there any bar jobs available and to ring some Turkish fucker who ran a pub in Nantes and ask him for references. Myself and Vinnie looked at each other the second they hiked out the door.

—So would I, said Vinnie.

We laughed so much Joan came in from the kitchen to see what was on the telly.

Cricket arrived live on the satellite from the other side of the world a month later so we had a lock-in. I saw Kerrie looking at me in a way you couldn't mistake for anything else when I rebolted the door after the last customer left. Kim came over and kissed me hard on the face. Vinnie called a taxi for Kerrie.

A week later. Myself and Vinnie postponed the clean-up and went down to the Mexican bar and restaurant on the Green where you paid clip-joint prices for mushy concoctions of chicken and chillies and at half eleven the King William punters came in to if you were lucky nibble at your meal and if you were unlucky fall into it.

The Kiwis from the squat wore tops that showed their belly buttons. They stood in a circle and clutched nervously at bottles of tepid Mexican beer with limes wedged in the mouth.

—*La bamba* is Italian for the goat, Vinnie told me.

The music changed to something slow by Gloria Estefan and the crowd moved and pitched me into the middle of the Kiwis. I covered my embarrassment by dragging Kerrie out to dance.

—*Goat, the Goat, Goat, the Goat* is a very peculiar chorus, isn't it, boss, Vinnie was shouting.

I took Kerrie up to see Kaya sleeping when the Mexican closed. She gently removed the thumb from Kaya's mouth because seemingly that can push their teeth out when they're that age and they end up having to wear a brace and girls hate having to wear a brace, Paul, because it makes them stand out and we're sensitive about those sorts of things. I put my arms around her very clumsily. She moved away.

—Paul, what are you doing? Just because I work for you doesn't mean you can just pick me up in a bar and bring me back here for a one-night stand.

—It's not like that.

Though what it was like I could not say.

—I don't know. Kim told me she thought you were looking for someone to love you.

She pressed my hand against the hard perfect nub of flesh above her waist which showed she had definitely not been delivered by the alcoholic midwife who years ago in Rathbawn had been paid in drink and left the population with navels you could hang your hat on.

—What do you call a hula hoop with spikes? A navel destroyer.

The joke was the first thing into my mind the next morning when the Samurai alarm clock woke the pair of us. The scent of tabasco sauce made a curtain across the room. Kerrie swung herself out of bed and looked out the window. I propped an extra pillow under my head and looked at her tanned body while she stood there. Something about her nakedness showed she thought this was a place she belonged.

I tried not to but that moment for the first time in a long time I thought if toothpaste prevented tooth decay it was a pity they hadn't developed it into an ointment you could rub all over your body.

You could put it on with a yard brush.

And the final nuclear holocaust would have been a disaster altogether at that point in time.

—Hello.

—Hello, Vinnie. The pants of you, you're not fit, you cunt. You'll get a heart attack.

—You'll have to put in one of those stair lifts. How is everything going?

—I'm having a ball. Gee, it's good to be back in magical, mystical Ireland.

—You sound well. Like seriously you do, boss. You sound settled. You'll be back soon?

—I will. Don't forget the quiz competition starts next week and the bus has to be booked now for the beano to Brighton. Ye're keeping it ticking over anyways?

—Like a time bomb under Mountbatten's boat.

—Honestly, you know, if I loved men I'd love you.

—You soppy shite, hurry up and get back.

—'Bye 'bye, baby.

—Baby, 'bye 'bye.

There should have been fewer things bugging me on my way back to Donoghue's. But there was a big extra one. Where was Bumper? It wasn't just like he hadn't turned up yet. It was like he actively wasn't there. I had a hunch I wouldn't see him again that day. It bothered me. I couldn't kill the Lone Wolf without seeing Bumper first.

Kaya and the two boys were squirting each other with water pistols. Richie Fee had come into the pub with a box of them shoved under his jacket after a trip down to Carolan's Joke Shop. Theresa said she was fond of the colour green so she bought three and haggled a spud gun and two ping-pong paddles out of him as part of the deal.

—We'll have another one, Theresa.

—Whatever you say, Paul. I'll just go out to the sink and fill Kaya's gun.

I loved pubs even before I was an alcoholic. It's why the only thing I've ever been good at in my life is running them. What I love most is how they have their own light. They carry it inside them. That light is different in every pub. Because of the way it bounces off the walls and streams in through the doors. Because of the different shapes of windows and the tint the light takes off the glass and the amount of smoke and dust that seeps into it. And the way it changes like it had in Donoghue's where Kaya's tired head was in my arms. The corn-row gone and her hair tied up with an Alice band. Mam probably thought that was more appropriate. As if she had a clue about Kaya or knew anything about the sort of person my daughter was. I knew she didn't.

Because my daughter was going to be different. She wasn't Tracey nor she wasn't Liz. She wasn't me neither. And if she kept out of Rathbawn and stayed in London she never would be. I thought that and finally Kerrie's face did come back to me.

Time is different too in a pub. The hands on the clock are only black spiders doing meaningless laps. Little crystalline slivers of ice in the Jemmy gave me joy in my heart, kept me singing.

—What are you thinking about, Paul?

—Nothing.

—You know what thought did, said Kaya, and the three nippers burst into giggles.

Something sour seeped into my mouth. It wasn't the whiskey. It was a question.

Why?

Kerrie probably asked herself that most nights even though no one asked her to.

—Kim told me she thought you were looking for someone to love you.

And Kim was sharp. She had a degree in archaeology which seemingly was a better one than Kerrie's which was in communications.

Kerrie might be able to have enough love for the pair of us. To make up for what had been knocked out of me by an unattended pram I hadn't even seen. Maybe what I felt for her came from her damp and sticky love overflowing on to me. Or I felt the same way she did but, because I didn't know, love reflected off me and bounced on to Kerrie so there just seemed to be twice as much love on her side.

I daydreamed in Donoghue's of Kaya. Her sturdy shoes bringing her up to the top of the Eiffel Tower with her school chums from Malory Towers. And some college somewhere and not a communications degree but an archaeology degree and the ability to lounge around second-hand bookshops like the one next door to the King William and pick up a book.

—Look Tristan, look Penny, Márquez, Márquez.

The sort of life that suited the softness of her face. Kerrie knew about that life and how to keep someone on the path towards it.

That daydream ran over and over again like a busted action replay as the day went down the plughole. One of the big newses came on and I didn't know if it was six or nine. Kaya's nose breathed little tired wet drops of sleep that made the hairs on the side of my hand quiver. I wondered if she would ever know that her father had decided to kill a man.

A commotion in the bar. The door slammed repeatedly. People rushed out into the street.

—Paul, there's been shots fired down the bottom end of Colmcille Park.

I didn't see Theresa and Kaya as I was running out the door. I didn't see anyone till I landed at the bottom of the hill. An ambulance and two squads roared past me to swell the number of people gathered outside our front gate.

Mam leaned against the garden wall and tried to console Liz. 0800 directed the ambulance towards where he'd kept people away from a bunched-up heap surrounded by blood.

Greer's front door was gone. Their windows were pitted with perfect round circles. Missus Greer was in hysterics. She swung a bird cage filled with the red splotch of an ex-canary round her head. A couple of people tried to get

Belinda Greer to sit down. Her teeth polar-bear-chattered. A large stain had spread down the front of her white jeans. Young Gerry Greer gabbed away to a frantic bluebottle.

—We were watching telly and then the window broke and three bullets went through the budgie and I knew it was gunfire from watching cop shows on the telly. And then we all got down on the floor and we could hear them battering down the door and I thought we were goners. And they saw Belinda up on the landing so they shot up the stairs and they missed her and one of them has this ape face on him and he's shouting how ya like me now motherfucker and going come out Kelly you cunt and I shout this is Greer's, Kelly's is next door.

Smart-Casual arrived. He put his hand on my shoulder.

—Oh, Christ on a fucking nine-speed racer. This is a pure disgrace now.

As if some etiquette had been breached and there'd be wigs on the green. Mam came over to hug me and say that that poor Richie Fee was only after coming in to sell her a couple of buckets dead cheap and she was after seeing him out the gate when the two lads came over and started larruping him. She thought it was a joke because one of them wore a gorilla mask.

Richie Fee's eyes were wide open but you could hardly see them. The swelling was risen on his face already. His head looked like it was going to burst. His voice carried deadly clear from the stretcher.

—And they kept saying we have you now Kelly, you're one stone-dead homie. Only the gun jammed when the gorilla man pointed it at me and he lost the head so they started hammering me with these baseball bats. Me hands feel funny.

He poked his arms from underneath the blanket. He wasn't able to lift his head up enough to see his little fingers weren't there any more. Two red stumps with jagged marks at the top showed where they had been. The medics couldn't seem to find them. The street lighting was gammy for that sort of assignment. I led Mam into the house. She hadn't copped what tonight was about. I made her hot milk and dosed it with Normison's. Then myself and Uncle Jimmy sat up and listened to the action outside where Richie Fee's brothers and girlfriend had arrived and were kicking and climbing up on the squad cars because no one would tell them whose fault this all was.

I knew whose it was. And I knew what I had to do in the morning.

Sixteen

Dead Men on Leave

It was going to be a happy day. The sun was an orange ball from a picture book where the perfect blue sky had little turned-down corners so you could take it with you. I wanted to get Kaya and swing her around in the air and tell her, yes, she had the right idea and the world was as happy as a four-year-old thought. And no worse than a four-year-old could imagine.

The white car shone like snow blindness. The drinks company logo scrolled purposefully along its side. Bumper leaned up against it.

—Top of the morning to you, your honour.

—And to yourself, Bumper.

—You forgot something.

He bunched three fingers into his palm, pointed the other one straight ahead and cocked his thumb back. He snapped it forward.

—Bang.

The Smith and Wesson was still in the bottom of the wardrobe. I locked the bedroom door and hunkered down for a couple of minutes. I hoped it might have disappeared but it hadn't. There it was with the two notches in the handle reminding me I'd seen it before. A well-loved friend, the same gun. I sat on the edge of the bed and loaded it.

I could shoot myself in the knee. Everyone would think it was an accident and I would get a few weeks in hospital before checking out and sneaking off to some place where nobody would know me. Paul Kelly. Knight of the Road.

Only I had this picture of Bumper arriving in with a bunch of flowers on my first day in hospital. Telling me this was all very well but get up on those crutches like a good man and go across to Abbeytown and shoot Cathal O'Hagan, aka the Lone Wolf. Because I knew Bumper knew who I was going to shoot. He might have known all along. It really didn't matter that much.

The gun in my jacket pocket made me feel a million times better. I doused myself with Joop. I put on so much that rivulets thick enough to be rivets rolled down my neck and puddled into stains on my collar. The sweat was beginning already. Chilled. The front door closed behind me at the second attempt.

In the name of my daughter and of my wife and of my brother's ghost. So shall there be an end. The one way or the other. Walkin', I'm walkin'.

I put my hand up to my jacket pocket a couple of times. I felt great now. The gun felt like a full wallet early in a good night. It was all I needed. Hey, you, are you trying to rob my pub? Well, suck on this, boy. Hey, Sean, you think you're so fucking smart, with your drugs, put your hands over your head and don't move. Hey, cops and everyone who thinks they're smart, don't even look at me fucking sideways or you'll get a bullet into the head.

The answer to everything. I'm telling you. Even Bumper couldn't take on a man with a gun or he'd be offski. Dead meat. Yes that is a gun in my pocket and I am very glad to see you. I could see why you'd never want to leave one of these yokes down once you'd carried it. You knew it made sense.

But Bumper didn't look at me anyways differently. Didn't he know I could just whip out my piece and blow him to kingdom come? Boom. Boom. Boom. Boom. I was surprised at what my voice said. It sounded like a squeak beamed in from a long way away. Radio interference.

—Can you not do it, Bumper? Why is it me that has to do this job?

—I'm known over there. It'd be too risky. Go on, you can do it, I have great faith in you.

The door was unlocked. The keys were in the ignition. I had the engine started before something occurred to me.

—Bumper. Do you know who I'm supposed to kill in Abbeytown?

—I do. The big kahuna. You'd never know but there might be a photo of him in the glove compartment.

Bumper shuffled off with his hands in his pockets. I heard a yelp and looked in the wing mirror. Captain limped past Bumper on three legs.

There had been a crash in Sheepwalk. The fire brigade arrived to try and cut someone out of a mangled Audi Quattro. Two cops stopped the traffic with one wave of their hand. A couple of held-up drivers hooted their horns and turned their car radios up full blast in an obscure gesture of pique. The super was telling an agreeing woman reporter the recent incidents in Rathbawn were unconnected and it was irresponsible to describe them as gang warfare. He went on about family feuds which everyone listening would know was shorthand for:

—The gyppos is at it again.

Funny how people reckoned the tinkers were savages for taking revenge over what happened to their relations. You were only a sound man if you killed for a bit of a flag, an idea out of a book in a Hampstead shop or the chorus of a song by Thomas Davis. Respect due to Thomas, original gangsta rapper.

I felt sorry for the super. There he was telling Anastasia Kilduff there were unlikely to be any more incidents and here I was speeding across to Abbeytown to make a complete hames out of his forecast.

Well, not speeding exactly. Not speeding at all. Still not moving at a quarter past ten. Much more of a hold-up at this spot and I would arrive at the Chieftain just in time to miss the Wolf by two minutes. I half hoped I would.

I opened the glove compartment. Twelve spare rounds, a set of keys to who knows what, a mock-up driving licence, four loose sticks of Dentyne chewing gum. 'Your mouth is fresh, your breath is clean.'

Two snazzy black-and-white photos. Cathal O'Hagan. The Lone Wolf.

Typed on the back in case I was too thick to take a hint. Good, well-developed photos. I had expected a cheap photo-machine job. Now I knew that was a stupid idea.

You could see the Wolf hadn't a clue he was being photographed because he was turned slightly away from the camera in both pictures. He looked like a man who would face straight on into the lens if he knew it was there. The first photo was himself and another man standing outside a pub in Talbot Street. They were sharing a joke and the Wolf was smiling but you could see he was thinking of something else.

He was on his own in the other photo. Carrying a *Sporting Life* and again not looking at the camera. He couldn't have known it was there. I was sure. He would have made a face at it or given it the fingers or done something so it didn't just make a blank out of him.

His face was handsome with a few scars on it. It wasn't as old as I thought it would be. I looked at it but there was no mark on it to tell you what the man had done. It could have been the face of any Northerner who comes into your pub on a Saturday afternoon and asks for a pint and joins in the chat and whose religion remains unknown until the Rangers and Celtic results come on. These last few years you'd reckon the Prods were the far more cheerful mob of geezers.

The cops waved us on. Another ambulance arrived. The force were in good form even though you could nearly feel the moisture seeping through those heavy blue shirts. One of them looked in my window.

—Any chance of a few oul free bottles there?

—Ah, you know you can't be drinking on duty.

The cop smiled, jerked his thumb in my direction and said something to his companion. They waved at me. The road was set clear for Abbeytown. I wouldn't be there in time. I never was in time. Lydia could tell you that.

Lydia. Shit. No fucking way. Lydia would not be impressed by this journey. She would half-nelson me with one straight look.

—Paul, what do you mean you're going to kill someone? Don't be so silly. Go down for a couple of videos and I'll ring the Chinese and we'll have an evening in instead.

She never really believed I did the battering that landed me in England in the first place. I wished she would get out of my mind. She wasn't helping. Lydia would giggle and throw the gun away.

—I love you, Paul, because you don't have any harm in you towards anyone. Come on, I've got these oils that are supposed to be top buzz for the well-being. Come on, just give me a long massage and we'll both relax.

She knew I couldn't just massage her for even a minute.

Which Lydia though? There was one as well that left her kid daughter in a pram in the heart of Junkieland and ended up turning tricks. That Lydia knew plenty of men who carried guns. She probably thought more of men who'd killed someone. Don't wimp out, motherfucker. Show Lydia Mark Two you've got what it takes.

Please. Please. Please. Please. Please. No.

Fuck it. Keep your fucking eyes on the fucking road ahead.

Think of Johnny. Johnny Mark One. Johnny crying when Christmas was over. Sniffling when Johnson's Baby Shampoo got into his eyes. A boy who thought I was the greatest footballer in Ireland. For my ninth birthday he spent a whole day doing this big painting of the Man. United team for me. Everyone in it looked like Arthur Albiston or Sammy McIllroy.

I'm sorry, Johnny.

I tied his fucking shoelaces, for fuck's sake, and put his shinguards inside his socks.

Which Paul?

Hello, Abbeytown, how you doing?

The Chieftain. Down from the power station. I'd never been in it. The sort of joint you'd drive past and say:

—I reckon there's a few tasty clients in there.

The crash hold-up left me thirty minutes late getting there. Half an hour for the Lone Wolf to drink his coffee. And munch his way through a Clubmilk or a Snack Bar if he was that way inclined.

Rap on the door. No answer. Second rap. Hard. Someone moved inside. The lights stayed switched off. A spyhole in the door. I stood right tight up against it so they'd have to open the door if they wanted to see who was there. Two bolts slid back and a catch clicked on. The gun felt a ton weight in my pocket but now I did feel like going in and blazing left, right and centre and maybe copping a couple of slugs myself. I think I knew in my heart of hearts I was too late.

—Go away. We're closed.

—How can ye be closed? It's half eleven.

—We're having a staff training day.

A catch in his voice as well as across the front door. I recognized it from my own early days in the pub game. But this kink wasn't going to be ironed out by experience. Not in the Chieftain.

—I'm a rep from the brewery. My rig is across the road there.

His eyes dropped to my jacket and he shut the door again. I wondered what the chances of kicking it open would be when it was on the catch. A cop car meandered by. But that must have just been a coincidence. You'd have needed a Sherman tank to break through the catch. It was probably the only new fixture in the pub.

—Aye, what do you want? We have rakes of stock and I'm not interested in any of those promotion nights.

—I'm here to do a check for the beer-line maintenance programme, to check the quality of your supplies and facilities.

—You'd have a fair clue yourself now about the sort of beer-line maintenance we'd have in this place.

—Sure you know the crack yourself. I don't check anything, I just come in and get you to sign a couple of things and you get a nice big framed cert to hang behind the counter and impress your customers.

—I don't think my customers would be too impressed by your fancy certs. They'd drink it out of a whore's boot, the same skins.

—There's a draw as well. Every pub that gets their beer-line maintenance programme certificate is entered into a prize draw for a trip to the World Cup for two.

—Who gets the prize?

—The boss man.

He did say my customers, didn't he? He did, yeah.

His hand went towards the door. It either hesitated or shook for a second. The catch came off. Little flecks of old green paint and splinters of decaying wood fluttered to the ground as the door opened.

—Come on in.

You'd expect a big man to be managing a pub like the Chieftain and you wouldn't be wrong. He was no height at all but he had arms on him like a Wheelchair Olympics champion and a belly that his customers would one day remember and say:

—Ah, yes, he was a young enough man but you could always see it coming.

Moist and worn eyes perched above the cracked red skin of his cheeks. They carried the questioning look you see looking over the bar when all that's in is men drinking on their own and frantically leafing through newspapers they've already read cover to cover a dozen times.

—Where are these oul forms you want me to sign?

—They're in the pocket of me jacket.

—Do you want a sandwich? On the house.

An irregular pile of ham sandwiches loitered in a dirty plastic box on top of the counter. I shook my head and realized that the Lone Wolf wouldn't have had anything in the substantial line to eat along with his coffee. If he'd been in the pub at all.

The manager waited expectantly with his paw stuck out. Great how people entered in any draw are already working out what to do with the top prize. I looked round. No threads left on the carpet, bluebottles circling a fan that worked in epileptic fits and starts and two increasingly familiar circles just above the fag machine. It takes negative action to produce a kip like the Chieftain. Four oul lads dotted round the pub drank doubles as chasers and looked straight ahead. Three empty cups of coffee on the bar.

I touched my finger to a small drop in one of the cups and put it to my tongue. Luke-warm. A beer mat peeled into layers to one side of the cups. A coaster hemming them in on the other side. Someone had been doing those little boxes where you draw a line back from a square and join it to another square so it looks three-dimensional. Isometric projection. In black biro. They'd tried it with triangles but it hadn't worked out. Someone else had been looking at the *Star*'s TV pages. You could tell it was a different person because the circle around *The New Adventures of Superman* was in blue biro.

—Have you got these forms for me or what? I can't afford to be wasting my time.

None of us can but he wasn't the sort of bloke you'd discuss that sort of thing with.

—Was Cathal O'Hagan in here this morning?

—What?

—Cathal O'Hagan. He's an old mate of mine. I was just wondering was he in here earlier.

—I never heard tell of anyone by that name in this pub. He must be a stranger. O'Hagan wouldn't be an Abbeytown name.

—He's a small fella with a Northern Irish accent. You'd know him if you saw him. Curly hair, sort of sunken-back eyes and three scars bunched together on his right jaw.

He knew him all right. The wet eyes blinked twice and he pretended he had to do something with the sandwich container. The mitts were trembling chronic bad so all he did was send the pyramid of bread and ham all over the shop. The smell of rancid butter hit me at some spot right in the back of my nose. It made me wince. He must have mistook it for something to do with fear because all of a sudden he got bould.

—I never heard of him. I never saw the man at all but I'm telling you something now that you wouldn't want to be coming around this pub asking too many questions because there's men here would bate manners into you quick enough.

The gun. I could have shown him the gun and seen how hard he was. I could have poked it right up into his nose and asked him if he wanted to stay bould. He had no gun. I could have taken it out of my pocket, cool for cats like, and shown him the difference between men who had guns and men who didn't have guns. That was what it was for. Instead I made for the door. I knew I wouldn't be back to the Chieftain to look for the Wolf any more.

—You know you're getting old when the guards seem to get stupider every year.

His shout came after me. I slammed the door. A shower of wood flakes showered into my mouth and hair and set me coughing.

The exact second I walked out I saw the Lone Wolf, aka Cathal O'Hagan, walking into the Hot 'n' Kickin' Rib Shack across the street. Five seconds later or five seconds earlier I wouldn't have. Chance but. Better not to think about it.

I checked the photos again just in case please God there might be a chance that wasn't who I saw walking into the Hot 'n' Kickin' Rib Shack. But it was him all right. The Lone Wolf. The Boss. *Il Capo di Tutti*. *Le Grand Fromage*. *An Taoiseach*.

The two boys standing inside the door of the Hot 'n' Kickin' wore House of Pain T-shirts. I knew what the story was even before one of them stepped out in front of me.

—Sorry, you can't come in.

—Excuse me. I have to, I'm from the brewery.

—Well, excuse me, buddy boy, but you mustn't be from around here or you'd know that we don't ask people, we tell them.

—Come on, boys. They have no supplies of booze for the

day if I don't get in now. I have to be in Cordrum in twenty minutes. They'll be dry all evening if I don't get in.

They looked at each other. The eyes a bit out beyond bleary. One grill hissed inside in the Rib Shack. All the staff gathered round it and tried to look busy. The rest of the place was like a graveyard. They hadn't bothered to switch on the lights over the other grills. If anyone knew what the brewery rep looked like I'd hardly make it back to the nice white car with the expertly executed logo. Executed. That's a good one, all things considered. Hey? Hey?

—We keep an eye on this place. I think to prove you're OK you should give us a few bottles as a mark of respect.

—No problem, lads. How would a crate of Beck's between ye suit?

—Crate each.

Number two nodded. I couldn't believe they didn't smell the gun.

—I just have to go in and see exactly how much drink they want. I'll be going back to the car then. It's parked across the road there, see?

Another nod. They looked a bit knackered. They let me go when I pushed past them. I didn't think they'd normally let a push go but it was early in the day. A quarter to twelve and not a child in the house washed. I heard the tail-end of a conversation about exactly what sort of drink Beck's was as I walked down the length of the Rib Shack.

It was a long, narrow spot. Like all those diners, rib shacks and pizza pie factories that sprouted up in Ireland. Your arms would nearly stretch from one side wall to the other but lengthways it was like a long hall into a big house. A blonde girl in a silly red hat dropped a lock of coins into the little jukeboxes sitting on top of the formica counter.

A lad with a ring in his lip tacked up witty placards on the wall. Those drawings of men and women that are supposed to be something to do with 1950s America though I can't imagine anyone ever really drew like that. Another boy tossed bottles of Bud up in the air and caught them behind his back. He was good. A lot of people are good at that. I suppose that means it's easy.

The Lone Wolf sat in the very last table. Next door to the jacks. A young one mopped the floor inside and kept an eye on him. The Lone Wolf paid no mind to her. He went through the racing pages, cross-checking tipsters from different papers against each other. I watched him for a minute. He looked at his watch but he didn't look up.

One of the bottles of Bud hit the ground. The crash was louder than all the spitting and roasting. The Lone Wolf lifted his head. He saw me a split second after he started shouting.

—Any sign of this fucking all-day breakfast at all? Who the fuck are you? This place is closed for the moment, get out to fuck.

—My name is Paul Kelly.

My voice sounded now like I'd wanted it to sound when I was talking to Bumper. I was floating away above all this. This didn't seem like I was in it. It didn't seem like anything. I put my hand to my jacket pocket. Boom. Boom. Boom. Boom. None of it was real. Those dorky posters and the music now turned up full blast so the Wolf had to lean towards me in order for either of us to hear the other.

I could see and he could see that his two minders had gone walkabout in the fresh air. I could have done it then. How fucking undramatic could you get? Even the walk down the Rib Shack floor was over so soon. The girl in the red hat plonked a massive plate of fried food in front of the Wolf. A couple of drops of saliva fell out of his mouth. He must have been ravening. That might have been what did it. I couldn't understand why you'd put a pancake with syrup on it next to rashers and black pudding.

—So, Paul, are you going to kill me?

His voice didn't hold up badly at all. If the Lone Wolf thought there was a void, he wasn't convinced he'd be heading there before the syrup stopped drying into the side of the black pudding. You couldn't get much more fucking disgusting. The gooey set of it. The Lone Wolf might reckon there were lots of voids.

—Paul Kelly, the famous Paul Kelly, are you going to kill me? You're not going to use that gun, are you? Ah you're not.

All of a sudden it seemed very hard to do. All of it. If he'd made a jump for me I might have been able to do it. I wasn't sure if what I felt was failure or resignation or just relief but I threw my hand away from the jacket pocket.

—I don't think so.

—I give you my word you're a safe man if you don't use that gun on me.

—I wouldn't be gone on your word.

He was smaller than I thought. But better built. Like there was too much energy compacted there to ever let him rest. He'd picked up a suntan somewhere along the way too.

—You might be right. Pragmatism is a more important tool than honour for a man of action. But now I know you're not going to kill me I have nothing more to do with you. You're no threat to me any more, we can let bygones be bygones.

—I want to talk to you. I want to know why all this happened. That'll put an end to it all.

—Sound.

The two girls behind the counter sang along with the jukebox for a second. They looked at each other, rolled their eyes upwards and burst into laughter. One of the lads frowned at them but then he smiled. The Wolf's minders hadn't come back so a few more customers trickled in. The Lone Wolf horsed his breakfast into him. He grimaced when he bit into the black pudding. The two girls stayed laughing.

Somehow this was my world and the gun just some Münch-hausen story no one would ever believe when I told it.

They say revenge is a dish best eaten cold. But so is quiche. And that tastes terrible.

—So what do you want to hear, Paul? Do you not think you should give me the gun? It might go off in your pocket and blow a hole in your chest.

—No. You're looking a bit rough. Were you on the razz last night?

—I don't drink. I've never touched a drop. Well, I did once in Portrush and I walked along the beach and worried about what it made me feel like doing. Never again. Pure waste of time and energy. I look better than you all the same. I know who sent you.

—Do you?

I didn't think I did. He yawned and I worked out how you could look that wrecked without jar.

—I've no quarrel with you, Paul. Not now. You know that.

—So what is it? Some Northern thing?

—Some Northern thing? That is such a fucking Free State thing to say.

They all did this. They went on at you about how inferior the last twenty-five years had made Southern Ireland and they ended up telling you that you had to visit Belfast or Derry (or Londonderry) or Portadown. And they meant it, man. The Wolf meant it more than anyone. He meant most things more than anyone. I wondered when someone had last disagreed with him.

—You're living in the Free State.

—Don't fucking come at me with that.

He ordered me some coffee and toast. The girl didn't ask him for money. Neither for that nor for his breakfast. He asked her to put some tunes on the jukebox for him. He went to hand her some coins but she waited for him to lay them on the table. He held his hand out for a few seconds before he gave up. The coins slid on to the formica.

I pushed my chair back just a bit from him because I could see the hunting knife inside his pocket. I patted the Smith and Wesson. Comfort if nothing else. Those dopey signs catch your eye somehow.

—When you're finished, pay your check and get out.

Someone turned the jukebox up another notch but we could hear each other perfectly now. We shouted over the music and drew quizzical glances from a granny in slippers sucking nonchalantly at a pinky concoction in a grubby glass.

—I decided in 1969 that there was only one way to take on British imperialism. They'd left us with no option. All power comes from the barrel of a gun. We took on one of the great powers in an armed struggle and you know as well as I do that it was a heroic battle we fought.

—Heroic, me fuck. What about teenagers blown up in pubs and kids killed in shopping centres and shoppers biting the dust outside Harrods? Every Irish person in England got shit for every bomb ye planted. It wasn't a war. If you were so anti-imperialist why were you blowing up working-class English kids?

—The Brits condemned themselves. They voted for Thatcher, didn't they?

—I voted Tory myself in the last election. I thought Major seemed OK and like Kinnock was a bit of a Welsh windbag. And I knew if Labour won all the money would be taken out of the country. And taxes would have gone up and I'd worked hard all my days in England and why should I have paid more tax to help out the Loony Left giving away money to their mates?

—You're only a fucking traitor, Paul. I'm surprised to hear that now, I had you down for being some ways intelligent. How can you vote Tory after what you've seen of the capitalist system?

—I'm not saying I'd do it again.

—The working class have to unite and smash the rotten edifice of capitalism.

—I didn't ask to be working-class. I had my own pub in England. I had a nice life. That's all people want, a nice life and to get out of the working class so they get nuff respect. Look at the estates in Rathbawn where they bought all the houses from the Council. There's some time for them. Whatever happens in any election or revolution or whatever, it'll make fuck-all difference for the people in the Park.

He shook his head and smacked his lips together and that was the closest I came to blowing his head off. Because he was being a know-all. And everyone thought they knew more than me from the moment Lydia drifted away.

But Lip-Ring came over and asked us to excuse him so he could sponge down the sign over our table: OUR WAIT-RESSES PINCH BACK.

—How can you go on about the working class anyways? You were at the same caper as Johnny, weren't you?

—It hardly counts. Rathbawn is a garrison town. In 1881 a member of the royal family visited the town and it was the people of the slums that came before Colmcille Park gave them the best welcome. Do ye deserve anything from us?

—You have a great long memory.

—Only 827 years long, Paul.

The two bozos appeared back at the front door and looked down anxiously. I felt a chill for a second because I knew I wouldn't be able to use the gun. But he waved them away. He was enjoying the chat. He could have talked all day.

Fats Domino's voice on the jukebox cheered me up. He made me look around and hope we were in a real diner full of bobbysoxers and James Dean. But the music faded behind the Wolf's voice. We'd been talking so long I wished I could think of him as Cathal. But I couldn't. Because he couldn't think of himself as Cathal. Not any more. Cathal was another dead shred.

—Sean Moylan, a great rebel leader, once defended his men for robbing post offices in the War of Independence. He pointed out that they put up with many hardships in the cause of Irish freedom and were entitled to help themselves. That's all I'm doing. I'm not a criminal. You're not allowed to even think that. I'm a left-wing intellectual. I learned all about politics and revolution when I was in jail, Carlos Marighela, Régis Debray, Herbert Marcuse, Frantz Fanon.

Boom boom boomerang didgeridoo. Diggi loo diggi ley. A ba ni bi a ba ni ba. That was what the list of names reminded me of. The fucking Eurovision Song Contest. Kerrie might be interested in them. But I doubted it. The names spooled on and on and on. I just looked at another one of those signs. It made more sense. It was worth believing in. IF YOU'RE NOT SERVED IN FIVE MINUTES, YOU'LL BE SERVED IN SEVEN OR NINE. RELAX.

The order to relax is one thing. Relaxing is another. Jesus, everyone tells you to relax. There were things I wanted to know and do before I got around to relaxing. There are always things you want to know and do before you get around to relaxing. But the immediates.

—What was it all about? Why did you have Johnny killed? Tell me that and I'll leave you to drink your coffee in peace.

—He was a scumbag. He really was everything I hate. If we'd been in the North, I could have had him kneecapped when he was a young fella and it would have done him some good.

I wondered did the Wolf ever listen to himself. A young lad came in off the street, grabbed a plate of chips from the table nearest the door and legged it out the door. Streaky black fingers crammed the Rib Shack French fries down his throat.

—We're going to try and sort out this area as regards the heroin end of things. It's stupid there's so much of the stuff in Dublin and so little of it down the country. I mean, there's good-sized towns around here, you could make a fucking fortune, you can't even imagine the wedge. Johnny thought he was a hard man but he was only a small villain. But he might have got in the way. He had to go.

So that was that. Johnny. The Lone Wolf. Heroin. Circles. Me and Lydia and Johnny and it all connected. A waste of time. Instead of London this was what I'd looked for. Confirmation of something else that could never be told. And Buddy Holly at the other wall not giving a shit and just keeping singing although now the world really was in pieces.

He was on form now. He waved up at the boys at the door. They moved out into the street. I could still have done it. Fuck the witnesses. Lydia would understand. But there was Kaya. There could be more. Fucked if I knew. Maybe it was just cowardice.

Snoopy Giff paced up and down outside with two mates who wore the same bad b-boy get-up. I'd need the gun after all. The Lone Wolf stretched out his hand. I thought there was a knife in it so I pulled the gun out of my jacket. He jumped back. A note of patient exasperation in his voice. A verbal pat on the head.

—Give me the gun, Paul. And go easy with it, Jesus you must never have handled one of these boys before. You never did, did you?

I shook my head. It meant agreement but you're never sure with these negative Irish questions. They always puzzle the Brits. But I was puzzled myself. I handed the gun over and looked out at Giff. All I had was a sensation of not caring any more. Caring had brought me no further than this.

—Don't worry about Giff. I've told him we're not

interested in you any more even though ye shouldn't have done that to his family. But Giff will do what he's told as long as I'm around. I've killed seventeen people and he's beginning to get an idea of what that entails.

The Wolf caressed the two notches in the gun and called me back when I'd walked four steps away. Another movie move.

—Just one more thing. I was going to tell you this in the beginning but then you had the gun and I didn't want you to think I'd done it because I was scared of you. I couldn't have that said, but we didn't kill your brother. Not me, not Giff. We were going to but someone else beat us to it.

—I think I still want to kill you.

—Don't bother, Paul. I'm going to die anyway. Revolutionaries are dead men on leave.

Giff tried to stare me out of it as I left but I couldn't work out what his eyes said. I just thought that once there was Cathal O'Hagan and it was 1968 and the rest of his life had not happened yet. Mam used say about the too hot summer when you get the maggots, then you get the flies and it all goes around in a circle again and will never stop until it is broken. I had a feeling Lydia was there with me as I walked out of the Hot 'n' Kickin' Rib Shack. Still expecting a bullet in the back and at that moment caring nothing about getting it. Johnny Kelly RIP. A sign above the rocketship bubblegum dispenser beside the cash register swung in the breeze of the opened door.

HAVE A NICE DAY NOW. Y'ALL COME BACK SOON.

Seventeen

A Pure Picasso Job

A steady stream of bashful street kids came to say goodbye to Kaya. She swapped Kangols, baseball caps and a pair of mittens for furry toys that had seen better days.

I gave the Samurai alarm clock to Liz and looked both sides of her ears when she asked me why. It was one less thing to pack, I told her. There was plenty of room in my bag. But what's the truth?

It was room I wanted to fill. I folded my clothes to the smallest possible common denominator so half of the bag stayed empty. I found one can of Löwenbräu in the bottom. It was warm and too sweet by this stage but I sipped it when I started filling the bag.

Johnny's collection of Rovers programmes. I knew Clinger wanted them but the guilt only lasted a second. An old Rovers scarf with the names of the team that won the League in 1976–77 fading fast. Two odd socks, one black, one white. A dog-racing card with four wins marked on it. Two old pairs of boxers, one with a polar bear's head peering towards the crotch. The dicky-bow discoloured by a soaking of Guinness. An old pair of plastic shinguards you'd hardly get your hand into now never mind your legs. But he'd been able to once. The bag bulged out strangely. Like an unmilked cow's distended undercarriage. It closed at the third attempt.

The train would bring us to Dublin that night. We would go back on the plane. Too much time to think on the boat. I had used it to delay my arrival home to Rathbawn. I knew that now. But there was no point delaying the journey back. I think I always knew that.

Mam was up. Raring to go. Perhaps secretly raring for me to go. The way we always long for what we are doing to finish and for the next thing to start. Maybe love is when you are happy to be in the time that's passing.

—You'll write this time, Paul. I don't mind what ye're at, I just want to know ye're all OK. But you should write, and tell Kaya to write as well, all her little pals will want to know how she is.

—I will write, Mam.

I would.

—And you'll come home from time to time, Paul. I'm not asking you to come back too often, just the odd time. On family occasions, it'd be nice to see you. There's no need for you not to come home.

—I will come home, Mam, don't worry. Honestly I will.

I wouldn't.

There was need for me not to come home. Father Muldoon could call me one more of our young people forced to emigrate. But people don't do anything. Not our people and not young people. Persons do things and there is something different in all their reasons and they don't add up to anything that means anything. No they and no we either. Except what is bonded together through love, though that is a word I don't know much about either. Why love? Who chose that name for it? You could call it offside or milk levy or the Magic Roundabout. Love is just some person's word.

Whatever the word was I would go back and see if it and me and Kerrie could exist in the same sentence. Kaya would be the capital letter and the full stop.

I needed to think you can break up most of your old world and find a new one and that out there is the possibility of doing this for ever until like some radioactive isotope your life gets smaller and smaller and eventually there is none of it left. But at least it kept changing.

London was a different world. And there might be a different world again after that. Rathbawn was my first world. My track was on it and its track was on me. That should have been enough for the pair of us.

The barrier between me and Tracey now was a good one. Though we'd lost some of what we had when we were kids, it had been time to lose it.

—It was good to see you, Paul.

—It was good to see you too, Tracey.

—No, but I mean it. It was good to see you.

—I mean it too, honestly. I fucking do mean it. Jesus, Tracey, I do mean it.

—I mean it too.

Francie was painting his front wall. The young Boyles were playing hopscotch and arguing what square the stone was on. It had landed on the junction of three, four and five.

Francie left down the paintbrush and spoke like he was pleading for a lenient sentence.

—Liz was saying if you come back in six months or that, she'd be so glad to see you. She says you shouldn't think that people don't want you here.

I nodded. Liz was in her bedroom with magazines about soap stars and disaffected royalty scattered on the duvet cover. She'd tried to skin up but had given up.

—Hello.

—Hiya.

—How're you feeling?

—Never better, Paul. Ah, you know, I'll get through it, I always do. Once you say you'll get through it, you're made up.

—It's harder not to get through it than it is to get through it.

—Yeah. You couldn't make that for us, could you?

I did. I had a hit. Gammy enough. But not Bisto and not parsley and that's not a bad start. Liz's pupils darted around for a bit. She settled back against the pillows Francie had probably piled high for her that morning.

—Liz, will you be all right?

—I don't know. You'd know as much about that as I would. You remember what Uncle Jimmy always said about Tracey being like Johnny and me being like you.

The white on Francie's paintbrush held the sunlight like a fly-paper trap as he waved goodbye to me. Two Council men took away the corpse of Captain and swatted the flies and wasps already making lanes through the thin body.

I knew this would be the last time I drank in Donoghue's. I knew it would be the last pint I would drink. It might be. One more for the road. Because I didn't want the bottle of sherry and six Roche Fives of two nights before to be my last memory of the alcohol game. Joe stood the drink. I tried to explain how I wouldn't be able to buy another one. He shook his head.

—I understand. I don't drink any more either. I don't do a lot of things any more.

—I'll miss this oul pub. This pub learned me most of what I know about the trade.

—I wouldn't say that exactly but I think you're better off at that beyond than scraping around here. Do you think the town has changed much?

—I think it's changed a sight in some ways and not at all in others. But I can't remember that well what it was like, you know that sort of a way?

—Here's a bottle of orange for the duchess. I don't think any of us can remember what it was like.

—Or if it was like anything in the first place.

I didn't think Bumper needed saying goodbye to. He'd know I was going and would decide on the appropriate farewell. Theresa I wouldn't see either. Wouldn't and couldn't. I just couldn't. I sent her a letter that morning. The second it dropped into the postbox I thought of a million things I could have said in it and a million others that I shouldn't have. I asked the postmaster if there was any way of getting them not to deliver letters already sent. He looked at me like I was on drugs. Hallucinogenic ones.

Theresa wouldn't expect anything different. I didn't know how that made me feel. It was her life. She might have expected something different from me. But she wouldn't have expected anything better for her. I wouldn't ring Kerrie or Vinnie when I got to Heathrow. I'd just walk into the public bar with Kaya on my shoulders and surprise everyone. There was no law against it. The letter to Theresa said things about me being bad for people and not worth anyone getting involved with. It could have been true but I shouldn't have said it was her welfare that worried me.

Kaya insisted on packing her new toys herself and choosing the outfit she'd wear. Her only worry was the Alice band but she had enough cop to say she'd wait till we were on the train before taking it off. I told her Kerrie would have the corn-row back in before she had to hit back to pre-school.

—Wikkid.

—Nuff respect.

—Dad. Don't you say those things, they sound sad when you say them.

—Irie.

—Dad. Seven seconds to comply.

—Stylee.

—Dad.

A little white ball of a fist thudded against my knee.

—Respect due to your dad.

They haven't a hope of resisting your tickles when their ribs still feel like they could snap in the wind. Wouldn't it be great if you could solve every disagreement in the world by tickling contests? If I'd read Carlos and Frantz and Régis and all the Lone Wolf's storytellers, I wouldn't come out with such guff. I'd be a serious and sensible man like him. I might go that way now I was off the drink. Forty-five minutes dry and the strain of sobriety kicking in already.

—Dad. Can we come back to Ireland?

—Are you sure you really want to?

—Yeah. Ireland's funny. They've got all these different games and songs and everything here and different clothes. I'd like to come back.

Roots and all that. Nah. Don't think so. Not really. This was a foreign country to her. That was it. That's what posh English kids are into. Travel. Probably because they have a choice in the matter. Kaya had all these years in front of her. Finding enlightenment in India, going to Tangier and haggling in souks, backpacking around Greece and finding this absolutely unspoiled fishing village that no tourists ever got near, sniffing at package holidays and making her way into the Basque country and telling people how you didn't really know anything about Russia till you'd spent some time there. Nothing had as much power over me as the vision of

Kaya's rucksack disappearing over cartoon hills and dales on her holidays from university.

All was packed. We stood out in the garden and watched a lob of young bucks chariot racing along O'Connell Crescent. It was that fine a day it seemed impossible anyone would fall. No one did. Eddie Clyne came to the gate. Walking. I thought he'd come to say goodbye.

Some major sadness had taken hold of his face and squashed the features up the way Rocky Marciano's fist distorts his opponent's face in the famous photo. He tried to speak but the only sound for an age was his teeth clicking and saliva being drawn back like a hammer from the insides of his lips as he prepared to break the silence and then found he couldn't.

Kerrie once brought me to the Tate Gallery. Women look fierce well in those dresses with Mondrian grids on them but I'm still not sure if those fellas could paint at all. But Kerrie made some sort of sense as we stood in front of a Picasso painting that I said reminded me of the Rathbawn Community Games art competition. And not the medal winners either.

She said Picasso had the right idea. Because you never do see a complete picture of anything. And all you remember are parts of glimpses and views from an angle and all the disjointed pieces that no two people ever put together in the same way.

It was a pure Picasso job when I looked in Eddie's eyes and I kept thinking of Elle the Body and how she had acted the first night we met and Clinger's arm going through the Imperial Hotel window. It all faded into the one big piece of truth and sense with no more angles left to work on. Like the Rothko guy just up the gallery from Picasso.

Eddie looked like he wanted to bolt. I was calm. So calm I was counting a minute under my breath and holding my right hand to my chest because I thought this must be the ideal heartbeat. Eddie spoke after twenty seconds and put me off my stroke.

—We'll go for a walk. I think we should look at the old haunts. I don't reckon you'll be back again so it might be an idea to say goodbye to them.

You can be as hard as you want but the sight of old places makes you feel some way like you did the last time you saw them. They remind you how you'll always be a stranger in the place you are now. And that it could be the ideal thing to stay a kid the whole time. The Pleasure Grounds, the five-a-side football pitch, the stream full of fish at the back of the Imperial Hotel where Richie Fee's brother drowned trying to escape from the cops, the wall outside what used to be the Dispensary where I hit my first hat-trick, the last goal a tap-in from six yards after Clinger rolled the ball across to me. Picasso's shapes broke up and reassembled as we walked.

Sense was being put on it. But it was the wrong sense. The wrong truth. Like the truth about Lydia. Like so many truths. Did it benefit anyone? Why do people always want to tell you things only to make themselves feel better? Pegging stones into the river. It was gas too. The end of it all and me and Eddie still tried to fling our pebbles further than each other. Then we tried to skim them better. But we'd lost the knack. They just hopped up once and disappeared.

—Do you want to know who killed Johnny?

—I have a sort of a clue.

I did. I didn't ask Eddie to tell me who killed Johnny. I didn't ask him to tell me why. He told me anyways. And when I looked away and started whistling he still did the old dog and held on to the bone and throttled the fucking marrow out of it. One hop. And then into the water.

—I killed him. Well, meself and Clinger did it but it was

294

my killing. It was my fault. I'm fucking sorry, Paul, I just can't hack it any more, fuck, fucking fuck.

—You can't even let Clinger have his own killing.

My voice burned the air like cheap red wine on to a stomach ulcer. How you like me now, motherfucker. Eddie didn't have to tell me anything. I hate knowing as much as anyone else.

Eddie was crying. I was crying. His arms were around my back. My hands were around his neck. I felt the way you do when you hold a little furry kitten. Hello, little furry kitten, I am your friend. But at the back of it your cute little neck is mine and if I squeeze you are fucked. Miaow. I hit him on the back of the head. He crumpled and fell into a pile of wet leaves. I could have sunk the boot into him and done anything. He just lay there shaking and waited for me to kill him. Back at the riverbank.

Me and Eddie lay on our stomachs by the riverbank the night Rovers won the Cup final and Duran Duran were number one for the first time. Looking at the invisible darkness in the water and drinking out of the same big bottle of Linden Village. He kept saying he had something to tell me. And refusing to say what it was. I thought he had some young one up the pole.

He snatched the bottle off me and tried to take a big drink out of it. Most of it missed his mouth and ran in streams down his chin, past his neck and across the white T-shirt that strained to contain his growing chest muscles. The patterns it made were like the diagram of an estuary in the Leaving Cert geography book.

—I love you, Paul.

—I love you too, maaaan.

—No, I mean it. I really love you.

—You're a real fucking hippy, do you know that? Kool in the kaftan, love and peace, maaaan.

—Don't be a fucking scumbag. I want to tell you this. I love you. I want to do things with you like kissing you and feeling you and everything. I want us to do them together.

He climbed to his feet and rocked from side to side. Holding on to the fence in front of the river to steady himself. He tried to look dead serious and dignified but his eyes kept beginning to close because of the drink. The two sets of eyelashes would just about meet and then his eyes would snap wide open like a Venus fly-trap in reverse. I believed him though.

—I don't want to hear this. Sit down.

—What are you worried about? I know you're not a queer and I'm not. But I want to tell you I love you because that's how I feel.

—Come on, I'll get you home. You're fluthered.

He'd fallen down in a heap on the bank then too. I'd run off and left him there. Neither of us ever mentioned that night again. Each of us prayed alcohol had taken away the other's memory of it. Until it didn't matter any more what we remembered.

I helped Eddie up. I went to pick two wet leaves off his jowl but he did it himself.

—It's not easy. But I can take it. It's Clinger it's killing. He's above in the house and he won't take a step out the door. He's there every day with tears rolling down his face and he's having nightmares and he can't look at me and he can't look at Bernie and he can't look at Sonia. Above all he can't look at Sonia. So he told her a couple of days ago and she said she'd get us taken care of. I found out she wanted to write a letter to you so I persuaded her I'd tell you and it was up to you what you wanted done then. She doesn't blame Clinger though, she blames me.

—No one ever blames Clinger.

—They're right. Clinger had so much time for Johnny. More time than he ever had for me that's gone through my whole life trying to keep him out of hassle. He wouldn't be able to live if people didn't look out for him.

—Why did it happen? Jesus, Eddie, you know how we all were.

—It was Gazza's fault.

—Gazza who?

—Gazza the footballer. Johnny turned into a right robbing cunt but me and Clinger stuck up for him against everyone because we knew that you have to get your crust some way. The Park, you know?

—The Park.

The two words said more than anything else I'd heard.

—But he got into Gazza in a big way. All the gear, same haircut, played the same way, never passed you the ball and strolled around midfield. He even put on a couple of stone. Then one evening we were drinking in Donoghue's and he said that Gazza was in with a married bird now, a fine blondey one, and he'd have to do the same.

—Shite.

—So he got in with Sonia. He was always a great hammerman and she was well into him. I found out and she told me she loved Johnny and she was going to leave me to be with him.

—So you bumped him off.

—Then he told her he didn't want her. He'd only been messing. Gazza had broken up with yer one, you see. Sonia tried to kill herself with tablets.

I held up my hands but Eddie wouldn't be stopped now.

—I love her. I know you think I'm a bollocks.

—I don't.

—I know you think I'm a bollocks. You mightn't think you think that but I know you do. I love her. Some people think it's me being the flash businessman with the blondey wife but it's not. If you're right in the heart you can't love that way. We said we'd give him a doing and tell him to keep away from Sonia. We met him coming home from the Dandy Diner and he copped when he saw us with the hurleys and the slash-hooks. Only he leaned up against the gate of one of those boarded-up houses and said he'd met Sonia again that evening and she'd given him a blowjob in one of the snugs.

There was a burrowing in the pit of my stomach. Uncle Jimmy's house had a steel plate at the back door but you could still hear the rats gnawing and chewing away at the wood and you knew they'd get in there in the end and maybe they could even eat away at your head and get in there and chew everything. Everything.

—Clinger went apeshit and knocked him on the ground. I think we were nearly finished leathering him when I copped that we'd gone too far. It was just our luck to kill him. But I'm sorry. I know how you felt about him. If it was my brother I know what I'd do. I'll tell the cops everything. We'll go up now if you want.

—You'll tell them nothing.

We stopped on the bridge and threw a stick each over. We raced to the other side but neither stick came out at the other side. Maybe they were too quick for us and gathered speed as they headed for the Shannon estuary and the Atlantic Ocean. I stopped at the gates of the new apartment complex where the Dispensary had been.

—Am I imagining things, Eddie, or was there a tap at the side of the old Dispensary where you could get a drink after a game of football?

—There was. You've got a great memory for that sort of thing.

—It was great. Do you remember when you'd be finished a game of three-and-in and you'd be parched and you could get this great drink of fresh cold water? You'd be made up.

Eddie's cigarette dropped out of his mouth. He didn't bother to pick it up off the smooth black slatey surface of the driveway into the apartments.

—Can you remember nothing? The water was bad. That was why we got stopped playing up there. The time eight of us ended up in the county hospital because we got poisoned by it. Johnny's health was never the same again. They reckon there was every sort of diseased shit in that water.

Eddie walked away from me when we got to the gates of his scrap yard. He stopped and spoke without facing me.

—You're sure you're not going to tell the cops?

—There wouldn't be any point.

There wouldn't be any point. Because there was no point. We were dying already. The Lone Wolf had it half right. Except it was all of us who were dead men on leave. It was like waiting for the healer in the morning at the monument. The minute you were healed it started you on the next session that would leave you in need of more healing the day after. There would never be a moment when you could say I am healed and that is that. There was only one way it was going to end and there would never be enough oblivion until the point when it didn't matter any more.

The Lone Wolf nearly found the words for it. But he knew the words weren't there. Words can't do that. It's not what they're there for. They skip us around it. The Lone Wolf's life was the thing itself. What he had done was it. He himself. Him and it sat at the Rib Shack table forking soggy pancake into his mouth. The Lone Wolf knew.

Bumper sat in his van outside Mam's house, playing a Smokie tape and chewing the bones from a Kentucky Fried Chicken. A party bucket lay on the footpath. I was glad to see him. He was about as real as it got. I wouldn't tell him about Eddie. It was over.

—Well, citizen.

—Well, Bumper.

—You didn't do it. You didn't kill the big man nor you didn't kill Giff. I thought you would.

—It's finished. I don't want any more revenge or anything, I don't think it means fuck-all.

—Sure I can't make you do what you don't want to. You'd be better off if you didn't think so much.

We snapped our hands out at the same time with some sort of ceremony. Bumper went to crush my fingers but then eased his grip. Something floated between us but there was no word to put on it.

—It's cowed you.

I shook my head.

—You're cowed all right. Every morning when I get up I tell meself I have to keep going and run over everything that's in my way or else I'll be cowed. Because the whole thing'll cow you if you don't keep going and stay in charge. And the day you're cowed, you're fucked. And Bumper Reilly will never be cowed.

I shrugged. He gave me a thumbs up and a jagged grin. I said the only words that sounded right.

—Leave it so.

Eighteen

Coffee Grounds

Go on. End it. Tell it. How Kaya's mother died. The woman I love died. Die is what she did that day. All the speculation about the might have beens of the this, that and the other of existence won't change that.

It was a Saturday afternoon. Kerrie had taken to staying overnight. I never asked her to even though it was what I wanted. In the morning there would be an odd silence as we waited till she made her excuse to leave. The silence would be broken by Vinnie exaggeratedly tidying up in the hall. Giving Kerrie the chance to throw some clothes on because he had to come in and ask me something.

Something was pleasant about that Saturday morning. I can't remember what it was now. Something uncomplicated. Neither me nor Kerrie were waiting for something to happen.

Laziness as much as anything else had us still in bed in the afternoon. We could hear Channel Four racing on the telly downstairs and the see-sawing of the door as Sligo Mick ran up and down with bets to South London Racing.

Kerrie had the blanket thrown off. She was sitting on my stomach and giving out to me because I wouldn't look her straight in the eye. Vinnie burst into the room and Kerrie just stayed there shaking with embarrassment and I launched a string of fucks at Vinnie who didn't seem to be looking at Kerrie anyway and I half knew what the crack was a tiny couple of moments before he spoke.

I knew it even before Vinnie burst into tears. Kaya started crying on cue in her cot. My wife was dying. She had asked to speak to me. Channel Four racing was turned up downstairs. Someone cheered a horse down the home straight. Winner all right.

Vinnie and Kerrie wanted to come up to the hospital with me. Then they wanted to call me a cab. But I wasn't on for listening that day.

The North London streets were wedged. Signs told me I was on a Red Route but I still stopped halfway up the Holloway Road and pressed my head into the steering wheel for five minutes. Those five minutes. No. They made no difference. But when you're saved, you still wonder if you should have drowned.

The doctor in Intensive Care was Indian and tired. He looked just jacked out. He spoke to me in a corridor and twice we had to dodge trolleys being hurried along the dented floor. None of those things are definitely true. The incidentals of that day are cloudy. All I can really remember is wanting to faint and come round five days later or else make some Country and Western deal with God to take anything he wanted in return for Lydia.

The doctor said Lydia had become conscious a couple of

times. She asked them to contact me the first time. The second time she asked them again.

—Are you estranged from your wife?

—I have been for a couple of years, yeah. What's wrong with her? Will she die? Will she live? Fuck it, doctor, I'm just sorry about all this. About all this fucking shite. I'm sorry, I am sorry.

—She's taken a heroin overdose. It could have been accidental. But her condition is so run-down that even a slight overdose could kill her. She really is incredibly debilitated. I'm sorry but I think you might have to prepare yourself for the worst. Your wife is unlikely to regain consciousness again. I'm sorry.

That is how they speak. You think there should be some different words to show how different this death is. But there aren't. The same words just come out and sound like they're stale from everyone else's tragedy. You can have nothing of your own. I didn't look at the fucker. I looked over his shoulder at a sign on the wall.

CELLULAR PHONES AND WALKIE-TALKIES CAN CAUSE DIAGNOSTIC EQUIPMENT AND LIFE-SUPPORT MACHINES TO MALFUNCTION. YOU ARE REQUESTED NOT TO USE THESE ITEMS WHILE IN THE HOSPITAL.

I doubt I would have recognized Lydia if I hadn't been told who she was. She was curled up in the bed. The size and shape of her like those little white coffins for burying dead children. A tube went into her mouth. Another was attached to her arm. A heart-monitor bleeped away beside the bed. I didn't like that. They were defying something to happen. I didn't look in case a straight line would run across the screen.

The blue hospital pyjamas were ridiculously baggy on her arms. The arms looked like they'd been scoured with acid. No veins there. Just patches of clear white skin with occasional small bruises. A nurse who drank in the Horse and Groom told me it's almost impossible to find a vein on a junkie if they need an injection.

I knew then why she had asked them to ring me. Because at that moment all I wanted her to be was back alive. Just to be alive. She could be on the other side of the world if that would make her happy. Just as long as I could know the odd time that she was alive.

I got the real fear then. Lydia's life was winding down slowly and I could do nothing about it except wonder if there had been a moment when this had started. Some time and place where a wrong turn had been taken.

When her body shook I knew what was happening.

All I wanted then was her eyes to flick open so I could cod myself she had seen me and some understanding had passed in the gaze between us that would make everything all right. Some final settlement.

The next shake was slighter. More of a tremble than a shake. There wasn't enough of her left to manage anything as solid as a shake. Brown, grainy fluid with a tinge of green dribbled slowly out of her mouth. It bubbled on her lips. Dried blood from what remained of her insides. The nurse in the Horse and Groom told me they called it coffee grounds. I held her hand. The wedding ring had been sold long ago.

They said the only personal effect she had on her when she was brought in was a little photo-booth snap. It was crumpled and stained. Lydia holding Kaya up in front of her and smiling. They were both smiling. No photo of me. Nothing except that one shot of Lydia and a daughter who wouldn't remember her. I lost the snap sometime during the week. It didn't matter. I never looked at any of our photos again. I had Kaya to look at.

I walked into a pub down the street from the hospital and

ordered a pint of Kronenbourg and a double brandy an hour after Lydia died.

We were sweeping the floors in the Flock of Swans one of the first days we met. Me and Lydia. She told me she wore contact lenses. I asked what they looked like. She gazed straight at me and lifted her top eyelid with her finger. She plucked out the lens. I looked straight into her pupil as she did so. The soft plastic lens rested on the tip of her index finger. I could see the little drops of wet from the inside of her eye. It seemed like I was looking at something important and secret.

Someone closed those eyes gently with their finger as I watched a quiz show and ordered two more drinks. There didn't seem to be much else it made sense for me to do.

I hung on in the house after I met Bumper and waited for the last train. The six o'clock news said a man had been murdered in Abbeytown. He had been identified as Cathal O'Hagan, 189 Collins Park, Abbeytown. Someone stuck him with a sword and then dropped a bottle of Calor gas on his head to finish the job. The police said they had not yet pinpointed a motive for the killing.

That made me laugh first. Then I realized they probably didn't know which motive to pinpoint.

I didn't feel anything. Not relief or sadness or anger. Because the Lone Wolf only sort of existed anyway. I did wonder who'd killed him. It could have been Bumper. It could have been the Branch man. It could even have been Snoopy. Or it could have been any one of a dozen ghosts coming at him from over the Border. I don't think being killed would have fazed him. I kind of hoped Bumper got him. It would have meant a lot to Bumper. But, to be honest with you, it didn't make much odds to me who had killed the Wolf. Because he hadn't killed Johnny. I don't think I would have cared even if he had.

Johnny was surely dead now. And nothing I could do would bring him back. The Lone Wolf was dead and then on came an ad about getting bigger bale silage and that was the Wolf's innings for the time being.

I sort of felt sorry for the superintendent though. He must feel like a notorious bollocks.

Kaya bounced around the room the way kids do when they're looking forward to a journey. And then on comes the man himself. Jamie Knox. There I'd been, worrying about his absence from *The Leuuve Zone* and feeling sorry for the cunt, and that wasn't the way it was at all, at all.

—Hi there, everybody, Jamie Knox here again. Just a-getting into my second week on the drivetime show and a-getting into my stride. The wife doesn't know herself since I've been able to spend some nights at home.

Good old Jamie Knox. Not on the fucking planet by any manner of means but I felt good for him.

And then it happened. I swear. This sounds like I'm making it up. But I'm not. It just happened there in Mam's kitchen with Kaya sitting on the arm of my chair as the second song clicked into the third. It did happen. I know it did. I couldn't have mistaken anything else for it.

Bob Marley's voice and the chug of the start and the three women I once saw on telly shaking their hands to the music and the sweat rolling off him and their heads all tied up with these rags. And start. And start.

> *Stir it up little darling*
> *Stir it up come on baby*
> *Come on and stir it up little darling*
> *Stir it up oh.*

I knew something was starting though it didn't happen at once. It just built up nice and slow and after a couple of seconds there was just me and this radio and dead Bob's voice and the love thing itself coming towards me and surrounding me and filling the room.

> It's been a long long time
> Since I got you on my mind
> And now you are here
> I said it's so clear
> To see what we can do
> Just me and you
> Come on and stir it up little darling
> Stir it up little darling

I don't know what did happen. But I felt all the forgotten feelings. Like I was back in that room when we listened to the song the first time. Once I'd heard that song and pictured myself and Lydia moving slowly together and smooching. When she left there was no picture in my mind any more. Now I saw me and Kerrie as my dislocated heart got pulled back into place by this song that hardly lasted three minutes and had been written for the money by Bob, and him sitting in the studio perhaps ganjaed out of his tree sharing a spliff with Carlton and Junior and Marcia and none of them knowing or caring where Rathbawn was.

Words cannot say. Only these words and music. No. But close enough. To the love thing. That song and memory close enough to whatever it was.

I felt like I hadn't looked at Kaya for years. She looked up at me with her thumb in her mouth and for once I forgot to warn her about her teeth.

—Kaya, do you know how you got your name?

—It's a song, Dad, ain't it?

—It's more than a song, Kaya.

—What's more than a song, Dad? You mean like a CD?

—Your mother loved you an awful lot, Kaya, she loved you when she put that name on you.

The streets on our way to the railway station were deadly quiet. A few street-traders in the Market Square saluted us. The old Dutch hippy who sold birds that were supposed to sing beckoned us so he could make me feel mean when I refused to buy Kaya a canary.

Ozzie Small slept at the foot of the War of Independence monument. An expression of peace decorated his snoring face. I tried to think something about Johnny. Something good or bad or indifferent. But I couldn't. All I thought was that I knew nothing about him.

Kaya pulled at my leg and looked up to tell me she'd protect me. I felt protected. But it was a protection racket. She would drive a hard bargain before she kept me safe.

—Shoulderbacks, Dad.

—Come off it, Kaya, don't waste time, love. Shoulderbacks is too dangerous. I'll give you piggybacks.

—Shoulderbacks, Dad.

—Shoulderbacks it is then.

We faced towards the station with Kaya on my back. Everything behind my back would be gone for ever in twenty minutes. Home.

—Come on, Kaya, let's go home.

I loved that film. And I always wanted to use that line. I know no one can be John Wayne any more but do you really think I'm the man who needs to be told?

I would bring Kerrie somewhere. It didn't matter where. I would bring her somewhere the sun shone and let her know why I had brought her there.

Life could be as simple and as connected with magic as the cave paintings at Altamira. We could go to Altamira, me and Kerrie and Kaya. I didn't know where it was but it sounded like the sun shone there. Even in the caves.